Nutrition and Women's Health

To my parents, Adeline and Leon Reidenberg, who encouraged me in my own pursuits long before such things became fashionable; my daughter, Amy, who inspired this book; my son, Gary, who cheered it on; and my husband, Alton, who encourages, inspires, cheers and sustains me.

NUTRITION and WOMEN'S HEALTH

MONA R. SUTNICK, R.D., Ed.D.

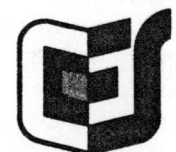

George F. Stickley Company
210 West Washington Square
Philadelphia, PA 19106

Copyright © 1984 by GEORGE F. STICKLEY COMPANY

ISBN #89313-041-9   LCC #84-050-690

All Rights reserved. No part of this book may be reproduced or used in any form or by any means—graphic, electronic, or mechanical, including photocopying, recording, taping, or information storage and retrieval systems—without permission from the publisher.

Manufactured in the United States of America; Published by the George F. Stickley Company, 210 W. Washington Square, Philadelphia, PA 19106.

CONTENTS

Preface .... *vii*

PART 1——THE BASICS: ESSENTIAL NUTRIENTS   **1**
   1 Carbohydrates 3
   2 Fats 11
   3 Proteins 19
   4 Vitamins 25
   5 Minerals 35
   6 Water 45

PART 2——WOMEN THROUGH THE LIFE CYCLE   **47**
   7 The Adolescent Woman 49
   8 The Adult Woman 57
   9 The Pregnant Woman and Nursing Mother ... 65
  10 The Aging Woman 79

PART 3——NUTRITION OF WOMEN WITH SPECIAL INTERESTS   **85**
  11 The Athletic Woman 87
  12 The Weight-Conscious Woman 93
  13 The Vegetarian Woman 107
  14 The Woman in the Food Market 115
  15 The Woman at Home 127
  16 The Woman Away from Home 145

Index *153*

Acknowledgments

Writing a book is an essentially solitary endeavor. In writing this book, however, my solitude was tempered by friends and colleagues who gave of their time, shared their expertise and offered their encouragement. I am grateful to them. Three women reviewed the entire manuscript; I am most deeply indebted to Miriam Diamond, Terry Heller and Amy Sutnick. Dorothy Barbo, Barbara Jacobs and Althea Zanecosky each gave me a generous measure of her specialized knowledge. Barbara, Althea and Brearley Karsch, Molly Kellogg, Leslie Piven, Julie Reidenberg, Norma Rosenberg and Marjorie Scharf read, commented on and enabled me to improve portions of the book. To them, too, I extend my thanks.

I have often read, in other books, acknowledgment of the patience and support of editors and publishers. George and Margot Stickley have shown me why, for which I thank them.

My family has been a wellspring of encouragement and enthusiasm. The dedication of this book to them is richly deserved for each one has played a role in its inception and completion. I must, in addition, express special appreciation to my daughter, Amy. She has served energetically, honestly and skillfully as my sounding-board, editor, critic and friend. It is a joy for me to thank her.

Preface

This is a book about food, the nutrients food provides, how the body uses these nutrients, and how people obtain nutrients by choosing and eating a variety of foods. It is also a book for and about women, and is concerned with their particular physiology and needs.

While everyone must eat in order to have the raw materials for all of the body's processes, women have special needs and interests related to nutrition and health. In their traditional roles of nurturers, wives, and mothers, women are concerned with nourishing their families as well as themselves. In their childbearing years and during pregnancy and lactation, women have special nutritional requirements. As they join the work force in increasing numbers, women are eating more meals away from home and want to be sure that their choices contribute to their good health. As consumers, women want to know about the products they purchase and how to get the best value for their money. And as the women's health movement has demonstrated, women are learning more about themselves and assuming more responsibility for their own health.

For all of these women, this book is designed to provide information about nutrition which will enable them to apply their knowledge toward choosing good food and planning good diets. Part I surveys the major classes of nutrients: carbohydrates, fats, protein, vitamins, minerals, and water. Each chapter explains what the nutrients are and how they function in the body, and lists food sources for each.

Part II examines the particular nutritional needs of women as they move through the life cycle, from adolescence through the childbearing years and into older age. Chapter 9 describes the special needs of pregnant women and nursing mothers.

Women with special interests are the subject of Part III. Nutrition is related to fitness for the athletic woman. Chapter 12 on the weight-conscious woman begins with basic information on energy balance and offers practical advice for women who want to lose or gain weight. Guidelines for obtaining sufficient protein, vitamins, and minerals from sources other than animal products are offered in Chapter 13 for the vegetarian woman.

A practical approach to nutrition is stressed throughout the book. In Part IV this approach is focused on the application of nutrition information to purchasing food in the supermarket, planning and preparing meals at home, and selecting food in restaurants.

It is the author's hope that this book will contribute to women's understanding of nutrition and encourage them to take an active role in promoting good health.

PART 1
The Basics: Essential Nutrients

1
CARBOHYDRATES

Bread and potatoes, cake and candy are the foods that come to mind when carbohydrates are mentioned, and these are good examples of two classes of carbohydrates, *starches* and *sugars*. Sugars and starches are important to us as a source of energy. For much of the world's population, carbohydrates provide up to 80 or 90 per cent of the total caloric (energy) intake. In the United States, we get about 45 to 50 per cent of our calories from carbohydrates.

Both sugars and starches are made up of simple sugars or monosaccharides (from the Greek words for "one" and "sugar"). Familiar monosaccharides are glucose, or blood sugar, the form in which sugar circulates in and is used by the body for energy, and fructose, or fruit sugar, the form commonly found in fruits, vegetables, and honey. When glucose and fructose are chemically joined they form the disaccharide ("two sugars"), sucrose, which is ordinary table sugar from sugar cane or beets. Milk sugar, lactose, is another disaccharide which is part of most people's everyday diets.

In addition to forming disaccharides, simple sugar units can link together in long, complex chains to become starches. When you eat starches, the digestive process breaks them down to simple sugars; it is in this form that starches are absorbed and utilized by the body. In plants monosaccharides can also be linked to each other in a way that the digestive system can't break down. These carbohydrates, known as fiber, move through the intestine without being digested.

The role of carbohydrates

The major function of carbohydrates is to provide energy. Once eaten, sugars and starches are easily digested and absorbed.* Sugars are generally absorbed and enter the blood stream rapidly because they don't need to be changed very much. Starches require more time for digestion, so are absorbed more slowly. Even the form in which the carbohydrate is eaten can make a difference. The sugar in apple juice, for example, is absorbed more rapidly than the sugar in a whole apple. And the carbohydrate from a food like bread or cereal is absorbed more gradually and "stays with you" longer than the sugar added to coffee or in a soft drink. After the sugar is absorbed, it can either be used immediately for energy or, if more is available than is needed, it can be saved for future use. Small amounts can be converted to glycogen, a kind of starch which is stored in the liver and muscles. These tissues can hold only about 300-400 grams (less than a pound) of glycogen. Once that limit is reached, additional carbohydrate is converted to fat for storage.

While the body can get the energy it needs from fat or protein as well as carbohydrate, it is necessary to have some carbohydrate in the diet each day. This is because carbohydrates do more than supply energy. Glucose is also broken down in the cells to provide products which are needed for normal fat utilization. Without sufficient carbohydrate, fats cannot be metabolized completely and ketones, substances formed during fat metabolism, build up to abnormal levels. "Sufficient carbohydrate" means some 40 to 60 grams, the amount you would get from two slices of bread, a half-cup of orange juice, and an apple.

Fiber

Fiber has no nutritional value in the sense of providing raw material for metabolism, and for a long time nutritionists con-

---

* Lactose is sometimes an exception to this general statement. There is an enzyme, lactase, in the intestines which breaks lactose into its monosaccharides, glucose and galactose. Babies all have high levels of lactase but in some people the amount of the enzyme decreases as they grow up.As this happens, they lose the ability to digest lactose and find that drinking milk gives them bellyaches, cramps or diarrhea. Individuals who cannot tolerate large amounts of milk may be able to drink small quantities, up to a cup. They may also be able to take fermented milk products such as yogurt or buttermilk.

sidered it of little or no importance. In the early 1970s, however, researchers compared diets and diseases occurring in African and American and western European populations. They found that the Africans had lower rates of several diseases, including colon cancer, diverticulitis (an intestinal disorder), hemorrhoids, gallstones, diabetes, and atherosclerosis. Their diets contained more carbohydrate, more fiber and less fat and protein than found in the western diets. Although an association of this type does not prove cause and effect, the surveys did focus new attention on the role of fiber in the diet and research on the subject is continuing.

What seems clear today is that a diet which includes a liberal amount of fiber promotes normal intestinal function. It may also help individuals with diabetes to control their disease and to decrease the risk of atherosclerosis and cancer of the colon. Foods which are good sources of fiber are whole grains, nuts, legumes, and fruits and vegetables, foods which are good sources of vitamins and minerals as well. A word of caution should be added. With fiber, as with many nutrients, *more* isn't always better. Fiber can react in the intestine with minerals such as calcium, iron and zinc to interfere with the absorption of the minerals. In practice, that means that eating whole grain rather than refined cereal products, and enjoying salads and generous servings of fresh fruits and vegetables is a good idea but loading up on purified bran and similar products may not be.

Nutritional value

We know that carbohydrate's value in nutrition is to provide energy. If the carbohydrate is eaten as fruits, vegetables, or enriched or whole grain cereals, then the foods are also a source of vitamins and minerals, but in its pure form, carbohydrate is strictly an energy source. The energy value of all digestible carbohydrates, starches and sugars, is the same: four calories per gram. This is true whether the source of the carbohydrate is bread, potatoes, or oranges or candy bars, table sugar, or honey. The nutritional value of the food depends on what it contains *in addition to* the carbohydrate.

At this point a word about a few particular sweets is in order. White sugar, brown sugar, honey and molasses are all essentially forms of sugar. The major differences among them are appearance and flavor, not nutritive value. It is true that brown sugar and molasses contain some iron and calcium and that these are important nutrients, but the quantities of them are minute. Table 1:1 shows the amounts of minerals in these sweeteners compared to some other foods. As a practical matter, choose sweeteners according to your taste preference, and be moderate in your use of any of them.

Dental caries

Another point of concern about carbohydrates is their role in the development of dental caries, or cavities. Everyone has some bacteria living in the mouth on the teeth. When sugars are eaten, some stick to the teeth where the bacteria can eat their share. Some of these bacteria convert the sugar into acid which is released on the surface of the teeth. This acid, in time, eats away at the tooth and a cavity is formed. Dental scientists are actively researching the ways in which different foods and different sources of carbohydrate affect the teeth, but the problem is a complex one. The effect of any food item may vary, depending on the form in which it is eaten; whether it is eaten alone or with other foods and beverages, or before or after other foods.

Table 1:1. Iron Content of Selected Sweeteners and Other Foods

Food (serving size)	Iron (milligrams)	Calories
White sugar, 1 tablespoon	—	45
Dark brown sugar, 1 tablespoon	0.4	50
Molasses, 1 tablespoon	0.4	50
Honey, 1 tablespoon	0.1	60
Peas, ½ cup	1.2	55
Broccoli, 1 stalk	0.8	25
Tomato juice, ½ cup	1.1	20
Whole wheat or enriched bread, 1 slice	0.5	55
Peanut butter, 2 tablespoons	0.6	170
Tuna fish, ½ cup	1.5	160
Lean beef, 3½ ounces	4.0	200
Egg, 1 medium	1.1	80

What can be said with certainty is that sugar from any source can be converted to acid and that the acid can remain on the teeth for twenty minutes or more. Eating a food high in fat and protein, such as nuts or cheese, may hasten the elimination of the acid, but as soon as more carbohydrate is eaten the process begins anew. To help prevent cavities, then, the best strategy is to limit the number of times that carbohydrates are eaten during the day. This doesn't require restricting foods at meals, rather, it means avoiding frequent or long-drawn-out sweet snacks. (A sweet beverage sipped over a long time keeps acid on the teeth longer than the same drink finished rapidly.) Other measures which will promote good oral health include oral hygiene - daily brushing and flossing to keep the mouth clean and reduce the number of bacteria - and proper fluoride intake, which will be discussed in Chapter 5.

Sugar consumption

How much sugar do Americans consume? The average is roughly two pounds of sucrose per week for every person in the United States, or *over one hundred pounds* per person per year. Moreover, sweeteners derived from corn - corn syrup, hydrolyzed cornstarch - are used in soft drinks, candies, jams, jellies, and other commercial products. Recent figures indicate that, in addition to our annual intake of over 100 pounds of sucrose, each of us consumes close to 40 pounds of corn sweeteners. About one-fourth of this is sold in the store as sugar; three-fourths of the total are sold in a vast array of products ranging from confections, cakes and cookies to beverages, breakfast cereals and crackers, and including frozen vegetables, sauces, and even chicken coating mixes. This sugar may appear on the label under a number of terms: sugar, sucrose, dextrose, glucose, fructose, corn syrup solids, corn sweeteners, and hydrolyzed cornstarch. It takes an informed and alert consumer to recognize them!

The woman who wishes to cut down on her sugar consumption has several options. The simplest way is to eat less sugar and sugary products; use less sugar - or none - in tea and coffee; and eat less candy, cake, sweetened cereals, and other sweets. Replace sweet desserts with fresh fruit. Snack on fruit, raw vegetables or crackers. Replacing soft drinks with fruit juices won't change your sugar intake very much but will provide more vitamins and minerals with the sugar.

Sugar substitutes

The other possibility is to use sugar substitutes or products made with them. The first fact to know about sugar substitutes is that not all of them are lower in calories than sugar. Two substitutes which are commonly used in sugarless sweets are sorbitol and mannitol. They belong to a group of compounds called *sugar alcohols*. These compounds are chemically related to sugars and have a similar caloric value. Sorbitol and mannitol differ from sugar in that they are not readily used by bacteria in the mouth so that they are safer than sugar for the teeth. They also are not as readily absorbed as sugar from the intestine. When a sugar alcohol is used in small amounts this slower absorption makes no practical difference. In large amounts, though, sorbitol or mannitol are not completely absorbed. The unabsorbed sugar alcohols remain in the intestine and draw in more water, causing diarrhea. That means that chewing sorbitol-sweetened gum or eating an occasional candy made with it is fine, but consuming amounts of an ounce or more can cause an unpleasant condition sometimes called "dieter's diarrhea."

Saccharin. There are other artificial sweeteners which have a zero or negligible caloric value. The most widely used of these is saccharin. Saccharin is also one of the more controversial substances in our food supply. It has been in use since its discovery in 1879 and has been in question for nearly as long. The most recent episode in the saccharin saga began in 1977 when the Food and Drug Administration proposed to ban its use as a food additive. The authority for the ban came from the 1958 Delaney Amendment to the Food, Drug and Cosmetics Act. The Amendment obliges the FDA to prohibit the use as a food additive of any substance which has been shown to cause cancer in humans or animals. In experiments conducted in Canada, rats born to mothers who had been given large doses of saccharin developed malignant tumors of the bladder. When the intention to ban saccharin was announced, there was a great outcry which ended only after Congress voted to place a moratorium on such a prohibition and prevented the FDA from acting. The moratorium was subsequently extended and remains in force today.

The dilemma with saccharin stems from the difficulty in establishing the risks associated with its use or, for that matter, the benefits it offers. Saccharin has not been shown to enhance people's ability to lose or control their weight. Neither has it been shown conclusively to cause any disease in humans. Many experts, however, are concerned about a major gap in our knowledge of saccharin's safety. Widespread use of saccharin in soft drinks and other prepared products began only in the 1960s; possible long-term or second generation effects might not show up before the 1990s. Furthermore, it is not known whether some individuals are more susceptible than others to effects of saccharin or how it can interact with other substances in the environment. Put simply, saccharin has not been shown to be beneficial, and its risks to humans cannot be accurately assessed. As in all matters of diet and health, each woman will have to make her own choices. It does seem prudent to avoid heavy saccharin use, particularly for young women, and especially during pregnancy.

Because of the problems associated with saccharin, researchers have been pursuing a variety of other non-caloric sweeteners. One which has recently appeared on the market is *aspartame*. Aspartame is composed of two amino acids, the basic units of protein, which are normal constituents of the diet. (One of them is phenylalanine, an amino acid which must be restricted in the diets of children and pregnant women who have phenylketonuria, a rare metabolic disease.) While the caloric value of amino acids is equivalent to that of sugar, aspartame is 300 times sweeter than sugar, so the amount used, and therefore its contribution of calories, is negligible. Aspartame has a pleasing, sweet taste in foods and beverages. However, it breaks down when heated, so that it cannot be used in cooked or baked products.

Alcohol

Although, strictly speaking, alcohol is not a carbohydrate, there are some similarities between them, and most alcoholic beverages also contain carbohydrate. Pure alcohol, like sugar or starch, is a good source of energy—and nothing else. Its caloric value is nearly double that of carbohydrates, seven calories per gram compared to four. Since beer and wine are made from grains and grapes, the fermented products still contain some of their nutrients but are inefficient sources of them. Distilled liquors provide no nutrients other than energy.

Each woman must of course decide for herself what role, if any, alcohol will play in her diet. For most nonpregnant women, moderate use of alcohol poses no problem. Some research even suggests that women, and men, who generally have one or two drinks each day enjoy better cardiovascular health than abstainers or those who take more than a drink or two. On the other hand, alcoholic drinks do provide calories without other nutrients - to say nothing of the caloric value of the nibbles that often accompany the drinks - a point of concern for some women. Alcoholism is a disease which is beyond the scope of this book, but any mention of alcohol in the diet would be incomplete without pointing out that excessive intake of alcohol is a problem for which professional help should be sought.

2
FATS

Fats and fatty acids, saturated fats and polyunsaturated fats, have been receiving great attention from scientists, the news media, and even in food advertising. Let's begin by defining the terms that are being bandied about by all of them.

Fats fall into a class of chemical compounds called *lipids*, which includes fats, oils, and other fatty substances. They are familiar in a variety of everyday sources: foods like butter, cooking oil, and meats; the oils that accumulate on hair and skin; creams, lotions, and grooming aids; and other common products. To a chemist, one feature shared by all of these materials is that they are insoluble in water but can be dissolved in "fat solvents" like ether or cleaning fluid.

Fats and oils

Fats and oils comprise the largest portion of the lipids we consume. Chemically, fats and oils are quite similar. Both are composed of glycerol, a kind of alcohol, chemically joined to three fatty acids. The difference as to which term is used depends on whether the particular lipid is solid or liquid at room temperature. Fatty acids are organic acids made of long chains of carbon atoms. Each carbon atom has the potential to hold two hydrogen atoms attached to it. If every carbon atom in a particular fatty acid is holding two hydrogens, the fatty acid is said to be "saturated." Like a sponge which is called saturated when it is holding all of the water it can carry, a fatty acid is saturated when it is holding all of the hydrogen it can carry. Sometimes the carbon chain has spots on it where two adjacent carbon atoms are attached to only one hydrogen apiece instead of the usual two. In that case, the fatty acid is not carrying its maximum load of hydrogen so it is called "unsaturated." When there is just one spot along the chain where this happens, the fatty acid is "monounsaturated." When there are more than one, the fatty acid is "polyunsaturated." The same terms are applied to fats and oils, based on their fatty acid composition. In general, the more saturated a fat is, the firmer it is. There are no totally saturated fats in nature, but there are great differences in the degree of unsaturation. For example, as any experienced cook knows, the fat on a beefsteak is harder than the fat on a chicken. When tested in a laboratory, chicken fat is found to be more unsaturated than beef fat. Vegetable oils, which are liquid at room temperature, are full of polyunsaturated fatty acids. One exception to this rule is olive oil which is mono- rather than polyunsaturated. When vegetable oils are solidified to make margarine or shortening, a chemical process which adds hydrogen to the fatty acids is used. The resulting hydrogenated vegetable oils are more saturated than the original liquid oils.

Cholesterol

Sterols are the second category of lipids which are important in nutrition. Sterols are very complicated molecules which do not contain any fatty acids but fit the criteria of being insoluble in water and soluble in fat solvents. The most important sterol in the diet is cholesterol. Cholesterol is a waxy substance which is an essential part of animal cell membranes but is not made by plants. Thus it occurs, in high or low concentrations, in all animal products but not in fruits, vegetables, seeds or grains, or in products made from them.

Digestion of fat

Compared to carbohydrates and proteins, fats require an extra step before they can be digested. Because digestive enzymes are dissolved in water and because fats, as we have seen, are insoluble in water, fats must first be dispersed into very small particles in order to be digested. The fatty acids are then detached from the glycerol and absorbed quite efficiently. After they are absorbed, fats also need an extra bit of processing to be transported and metabolized throughout the body. In order to circulate in the blood, which is essentially a water solution, fats must be linked to proteins to form water-soluble complexes called *lipoproteins*. Lipoproteins which contain a large amount of protein compared to the amount of lipid are relatively heavy and are referred to as "high density lipoproteins," sometimes abbreviated to HDL. If there is less protein and more of the lighter fat in the complex, it is a "low density lipoprotein," or LDL.

Sources of fat

Sources of fat abound in our diets. Except for skim milk and products made from it, all animal foods contain some fat. The amount varies, of course, depending on the specific food and how it is prepared. Careful trimming of meat can cut its fat content in half. Frying chicken, on the other hand, triples the fat level. The amount of fat in these and other foods is shown in Table 2:1. Notice that nuts and seeds are high in fat while

Table 2:1. Fat Content in Selected Foods

Food (serving size)	Fat (grams)	% Calories from Fat
Chicken, fried, average serving	20	55
Chicken, broiled, average serving	4	25
Potato, French fried, ½ cup	12	48
Potato, baked, 1 medium	0.1	1
Milk, skim, 1 cup	0.4	4
Milk, whole, 1 cup	8.5	50
Cheddar cheese, 1 ounce	9	73
Cream cheese, 1 ounce	10	90
Haddock, fried, 3½ ounces	6.5	35
Haddock, broiled, 3½ ounces	0.1	1
Apple pie, 1 slice	18	40
Apple, 1 medium	1	9
Club steak, untrimmed, 3½ ounces	40	80
Club steak, trimmed, 3½ ounces	13	48

fruits and vegetables, with the exceptions of olives and avocado, are fat-free. Dairy products range from zero fat in skim milk to very high levels in rich cheeses and ice cream.

The role of fat

Fats are the most efficient of all sources of energy, yielding nine calories per gram, more than twice as many as carbohydrates. Besides providing concentrated energy, fats contribute to the flavor and palatability of foods. They also increase the "satiety value" of foods: Foods containing fat stay longer in the stomach, keeping you feeling satisfied. Fats also contribute nutritionally by acting as carriers of the fat-soluble vitamins A, D, E and K and serving as the source of linoleic acid, an essential fatty acid which is required for normal metabolism. While the human body can make its own fat from dietary carbohydrate, protein or fat, linoleic acid cannot be formed from other nutrients. It takes just a small amount of fat to meet the need for linoleic acid; about four grams of fat in a day's meals providing 1800 calories is sufficient. Once eaten, digested and absorbed, food fat is either used for energy or converted to body fat for storage. In addition to being an energy reserve, fat serves several useful functions. It cushions and protects vital organs such as the kidney and insulates the body to protect it from cold. To serve these purposes, the healthy young woman's body is from 15 to 25 per cent fat. This percentage may increase somewhat with age, and it is only when fat accumulation is *excessive* that it becomes a health concern.

Smaller amounts of fat also serve other important purposes in the body. Lipids are an essential part of the membrane which surrounds each cell. Fatty acids are also needed for the synthesis of some hormones and of prostaglandins, a group of compounds which help to regulate body processes.

Dietary fat and heart disease

The role of dietary fat in *atherosclerosis* and heart disease has been the subject of extensive scientific and public concern. Atherosclerosis, a form of "hardening of the arteries," is a condition in which material called *plaque* is deposited along the walls of arteries. As the plaque accumulates, it narrows the space through which blood can flow. When this occurs in the small arteries which supply blood to the heart muscle, several things may happen. First—since the blood carries needed oxygen to the muscle—if too little blood is getting through, a portion of the heart may not receive enough oxygen for its function. This lack of oxygen, in turn, causes the pain in the chest known as *angina pectoris*. Second, a tiny clot may form in a blood vessel, be detached from the vessel wall and circulate in the blood. When the clot reaches a place in an artery that has been narrowed by plaque, it can plug up the artery and block the blood from getting through. This cuts off the oxygen supply to whatever part of the heart is affected, damaging the muscle and causing chest pain. In medical language, this is a *myocardial infarction*; in familiar terms, a heart attack.

Because the plaque contains lipids, especially cholesterol, it seemed likely that fat consumption and metabolism would be important areas for research into understanding and preventing atherosclerosis and heart attacks. Many studies have been done to determine the exact role of dietary fat in the development of heart disease, but the results are complicated and sometimes contradictory. In general, surveys comparing different populations find that higher fat intakes are associated with higher cholesterol levels in the blood and higher rates of heart disease. However, when researchers look at individual members of one population group, these associations are less apparent. This may reflect the fact that differences between populations are greater than differences among individuals in the same population, or it could be due to other environmental factors, identified and unidentified.

Another research approach has been to see how changing people's diets affects their blood cholesterol and cardiovascular health. Just decreasing cholesterol intake is not sufficient to make a difference in cholesterol levels because the body can manufacture cholesterol from readily available starting materials. To decrease cholesterol levels it is necessary to decrease consumption of both cholesterol and fat. To complicate matters further, it turns out that saturated fats tend to raise cholesterol levels while polyunsaturates tend to lower them. These observations are the basis for the many recommendations to decrease dietary fat and cholesterol and to replace saturated (animal) fats with polyunsaturated (vegetable) oils. At this point, you may be wondering why recommendations of this sort are so controversial. Unfortunately, there is no clear-cut picture here. Experiments have been designed to try to prevent heart disease by using low fat, low cholesterol diets to lower blood cholesterol levels. Some of the studies on controlled, well-defined groups of subjects have been successful. In other experiments conducted on large groups of free-living subjects, who are not so closely monitored, the results have been less clear. Along with such inconsistencies in the survey findings, the inconsistencies may be due to a variety of factors in the design and execution of the experiments, as well as in the actual causes of atherosclerosis and cardiovascular disease.

One effect of this difficulty in proving conclusively the role of diet in the cause of heart disease is that the consumer is deluged with conflicting recommendations for a healthy diet. This is due partly to the complexity of the science and partly to philosophical differences among scientists and health authorities. Given that the evidence linking dietary fat to heart disease is highly suggestive, but not absolutely conclusive, the issue becomes one of deciding at what point to act on the available information (see Table 2:2). There are those who want absolute proof that fat and cholesterol in the diet cause heart disease and

Table 2:2. Cholesterol Content of Selected Foods

Food, serving size	Cholesterol (milligrams)
Liver, 3½ ounces	300–750
Lobster, oysters	200–250
Egg, 1 medium	265
Beef, 3½ ounces	70
Lean fish, 3½ ounces	50
Whole milk, 1 cup	35
Skim milk, 1 cup	5
Butter, 1 teaspoon	11
Margarine, 1 teaspoon	0
Creamed cottage cheese, ½ cup	20
Dry cottage cheese, ½ cup	5
Bread, 1 slice	1
Fruits, vegetables, grains	0

feel that only then should the public be advised to modify their diets. The American Medical Association and a panel of the Food and Nutrition Board of the National Academy of Sciences have taken this position. On the other side are those who believe that we don't know when, if ever, we will have absolute proof; that the evidence we now have is convincing; and that reasonable changes in the diet are safe and offer the prospect of reducing the risk of heart disease. The first large organization to go on record in favor of modifying fat intake was the American Heart Association. In 1968 they recommended decreasing cholesterol and saturated fat and increasing polyunsaturated fat intake. In a second report issued in 1978, the AHA specified levels of 30 to 35 per cent of calories from fat (compared to the current 40 to 45 per cent) and 300 milligrams of cholesterol. Decreases in total fat, animal fat, and cholesterol were also endorsed by the Surgeon General of the United States and by the Departments of Agriculture and of Health, Education and Welfare (now Health and Human Services) in 1980. The latter did not advocate increases in polyunsaturates.

Dietary fat and cancer

More recently, interest in dietary fat and disease has been directed to the relationship of diet to cancer. Although still in a preliminary stage, there is evidence of a higher incidence of cancer of the breast and of the colon in populations who consume high fat diets. These data come from surveys comparing diet and disease in different populations, and from studies tracking Japanese immigrants to the United States. As these immigrants become acculturated and adopt American eating patterns, the incidence of specific types of cancer changes from that typical of the Japanese to that which is seen in Americans. On the basis of these observations and laboratory experiments, an expert committee of the National Research Council issued a set of interim dietary guidelines in 1982. While emphasizing that it is too early to publish final recommendations, the committee advised several measures, including reducing total fat to 30 per cent of calories.

Recommendations. It should be emphasized that these proposals are written on paper and not in stone. They represent current thinking of many, but not all, experts in several fields and are offered as a means of reducing the risk of heart disease and cancer. They do not pretend to be guarantees. They are, however, consistent. Whether the focus is on risk of cancer, heart disease or obesity, a lower fat intake looks promising. Although there are questions about the safety of higher consumption of polyunsaturates, there have been no problems caused by decreasing total fat intake from 40-45 per cent to 30-35 per cent of calories.

3
PROTEIN

Protein——its very name comes from the Greek term for "primary" and many people think of it as the most important nutrient. Actually, protein, like other nutrients, is essential but can't do the job of maintaining life by itself.

Chemically speaking, protein is the most complex nutrient. It always contains nitrogen and sometimes sulfur in addition to the carbon, hydrogen and oxygen that are also found in fats and carbohydrates. These elements are combined to form *amino acids*, the basic units of protein. Their structures are all similar, but there are enough differences to create 22 distinct amino acids. To make a protein, long chains of amino acids are strung together. A small protein molecule may have as few as 50 amino acid units; large proteins may contain thousands of amino acid units. In any case, it is the same 22 amino acids that make up the protein. To make the concept less confusing, try to picture a long necklace made of alternating red, yellow and blue beads. Now imagine the necklace with three red beads followed by one yellow and seven blues. Both are made of red, yellow and blue beads but the necklaces are different. And if you replace three kinds of beads with 22 different amino acids, you can begin to picture proteins. After the chains are put together, they twist, fold, and coil to create precise three-dimensional shapes that enable them to fulfill a variety of functions.

Role of protein

Proteins play a number of different roles in the body which distinguish this class of nutrients from carbohydrates and fats.

They are major constituents of all cells and tissues. This function alone requires a host of specific proteins to match the characteristics of each organ. Hair and nails, for example, are made of different proteins from the brain or liver. Soluble proteins are essential elements in blood and in the fluids both inside and outside of cells.

Another role in which proteins are ubiquitous in the body is as *enzymes*. Enzymes are the catalysts necessary for all of the biochemical transformations of life. The digestion and metabolism of other nutrients—and of protein itself—as well as all the other building-up and breakdown of matter that keep us alive require hundreds of specific biochemical reactions. The hundreds of enzymes that keep the reactions going are all finely specialized proteins. (Each of these reactions may require other nutrients functioning as cofactors. Some of these will be described in the chapters on vitamins and minerals.)

Other proteins are designed to do other jobs. Hemoglobin, no doubt, is the most familiar of the transport proteins. It is a protein bound to iron and found in red blood cells. (In fact, it is the iron in hemoglobin that makes the cells, and the blood, red.) Hemoglobin, as you probably know, carries oxygen from the lungs to every single cell in the body. In a similar way, other proteins transport other materials including copper and lipids throughout the body.

Certain of the *hormones*, biology's regulators, are proteins. Insulin, a hormone which controls carbohydrate metabolism and is lacking in diabetes, and growth hormone, to name just two, are proteins. There are other hormones such as adrenalin which are not protein but are chemically related to it. These hormones, too, are made from amino acids.

The diversity of protein's functions goes further. *Antibodies*, natural infection-fighters, are proteins. Special proteins in the blood form clots to stop the bleeding when you cut yourself. And when a woman is breastfeeding, she makes several different proteins which go into her milk.

Protein and energy

For protein to be used in these myriad ways, the proteins in the diet must be broken down to amino acids, absorbed, transported to the right place, and then recombined to make the particular protein which is needed. If, after all of this is done, there are amino acids left over, they can be used for energy; some are converted into glucose while others go directly to fat. The same route can be taken if the diet is too low in caloric value. Then protein is used for energy at the expense of its unique functions. This diversion of protein for energy isn't usually a problem in the United States, where diets are more apt to provide too much energy, but it does happen with very low-calorie diets.

Because of the priority of the need for energy, protein requirements can be affected by the calorie level of the diet. It is sometimes said that fat and carbohydrate "spare" protein by preventing its being used for energy.

When protein is used for energy, it yields four calories per gram, the same as carbohydrate. This means that replacing carbohydrate with protein, or vice versa, has no effect on calorie values. High-protein bread, for instance, provides no more or less calories than does ordinary bread.

The need for protein

Assuming adequate calories, how much protein does one need? Since the bulk of the protein requirement goes to build and maintain body tissues, the amount needed depends largely on the amount of tissue to be maintained. Protein requirements, therefore, are related to body size. Sustaining excess fat takes very little protein so that the requirement is really determined by the amount of the lean body mass, the muscle, vital organs, skin, bones, and other tissues which are primarily protein. While scientists are concerned with lean body mass, and can use sophisticated methods to measure it, as a practical matter we can relate protein need to "ideal body weight."

The amount of protein necessary to maintain the body is utilized for repair and replacement of tissue that is used up or worn out: hair and nails that have grown out, skin that sloughs off, and similar but invisible turnovers inside the body. Other processes can increase the need for protein. Growth means building new tissue and requires protein. The increase applies to a child gaining in stature or a pregnant woman supporting the growth of her unborn baby. The nursing mother, similarly, needs extra protein to make milk. Illness or injury also drain the body's protein and increase the requirement for maintenance or repair.

In contrast to these, physical activity does *not* change protein needs. An athlete engaging in intense body-building would need a bit, but only a bit, more protein to support the growth of muscle mass. But ordinary—and even most extraordinary—athletics have no effect on protein requirement. The hearty meals of steak and eggs long associated with training tables are a matter of cultural practices, not nutritional needs!

Protein in foods

The nature of the protein food itself plays a role in how much of it is needed to meet the body's requirements. This is because while we eat whole proteins in food, the requirements are for individual amino acids. Of the 22 amino acids, human beings can form about a dozen in the body. The remaining nine or ten must be obtained from food sources. These amino acids are referred to as "essential," meaning that it is essential that they be in the diet. The ones that can be made in the body are often called "non-essential," because it is not essential that they be eaten. They are needed to build tissue but can be made from the essential amino acids. A protein food which contains all of the essential amino acids in suitable amounts is a "complete" protein. In general, animal proteins are complete and are the most efficient sources. (The most glaring exception to this rule is gelatin, which is totally devoid of one of the essential amino acids.) Vegetable proteins, such as grains and beans, on the other hand, are more likely to be "incomplete," or lacking in one or more of the essential amino acids. To meet one's protein need from vegetable sources, then, it becomes necessary to consume a larger total amount of protein in order to get enough of the amino acids that are in short supply.

The usefulness of incomplete proteins can be improved by combining them to compensate for low levels of specific amino acids. Going back to the bead analogy, if you wanted to make a necklace of alternating red, yellow and blue beads and had a box containing many red and blue beads but very few yellow, you would have a short necklace and a lot of extra red and blue beads. But if you could find another box of beads that had a lot of yellows, you could make a long necklace even if the second box was low on blue beads. It's the same with amino acids. If one vegetable protein that is lacking in an essential amino acid is eaten with a second food that offers a generous supply of that amino acid, then the combination becomes an efficient protein source. Examples of this complementary use of proteins can be found in Chapter 13 on The Vegetarian Woman.

Table 3:1. Protein Content of Selected Foods

Foods, serving size	Protein (grams)
Chicken, 3½ ounces	25
Hamburger, lean, 3½ ounces	22
Haddock, 3½ ounces	19
Milk, 1 cup	8
Egg, 1 medium	6
Cottage cheese, ½-cup	15
Cheddar cheese, 1 ounce	7
Cream cheese, 1 ounce	2
Peanut butter, 2 tablespoons	8
Potato, 1 medium	3
Bread, 1 slice	2
Apple, 1 medium	0.3

Protein requirement. In making recommendations about protein intake, experts in the United States assume that people are eating a mixed diet which includes animal foods. Under these circumstances, an intake of 0.8 grams of protein per kilogram, or 0.37 grams per pound, of ideal body weight is considered desirable. In everyday terms, this means that a woman who weighs 120 pounds ought to eat 44 grams of protein each day. Forty-four grams of protein would be provided by eight ounces (1 cup) of milk, three-and-a-half ounces of chicken and two slices of bread, or by a half-cup of cottage cheese and a half-cup of tuna fish. Table 3:1 lists the amount of protein in servings of a variety of foods.

Extra protein

Clearly, most Americans eat more protein than is required. Fortunately, it is possible to maintain good health over a wide range of protein intakes; and eating more than is absolutely necessary is harmless for healthy people.

There are, however, a couple of cautions to consider before going all-out for a high protein diet, especially a high animal protein diet. For one thing, there is the energy value of protein foods. While protein itself is good for four calories per gram, egg white is virtually the only naturally occurring source of pure protein. Other animal sources, skim milk excepted, all contain fat as well, and sometimes large amounts of fat. An average 3-ounce hamburger has 22 grams of protein (half of a full day's allowance) and 15 grams of fat. That translates into 88 calories from protein and 135 calories from fat. The bun, by the way, yields 90 calories, mostly from complex carbohydrate. The significance of these numbers for any woman depends on her total diet and how each food fits into it. They do illustrate how high-protein foods contribute to the calorie level, as well as the futility of eating the meat and leaving the roll.

High levels of protein may also affect calcium balance by increasing the loss of calcium from the body. While more research is needed in this area, it has been shown that increasing the amount of protein in the diet results in more calcium being excreted in the urine. This is of special concern to women because the loss of calcium can lead to osteoporosis, a disease of bone which occurs most often in postmenopausal women. (There is a full discussion of osteoporosis in Chapter 10, The Aging Woman.)

4
VITAMINS

Back in 1912 scientists thought that there was a single amine, a substance similar to protein, that was vital to life. They called this substance, this vital amine, *vitamin*. Today we know that there are many, not just one, of these essential compounds and that they fit into various classes of chemicals; nonetheless, the name has stuck and we still speak of vitamins.

Vitamins are defined as essential dietary substances which cannot be made in the body and which are required by the body in very small amounts. They were given names according to the sequence in which they were discovered. First there was thought to be one vitamin. Then it was found that part of this vitamin was soluble in water and part soluble in fat and fat solvents. The fat-soluble portion was called vitamin A and the water-soluble part vitamin B. Then came another water-soluble vitamin, designated C, followed by fat-soluble vitamin D. When it turned out that vitamin B was really a cluster of compounds they were given numbers, B1, B2, and so on. As the chemistry of the vitamins was unraveled, names were attached to them so that today we use the name and the original letter interchangeably for ten of the vitamins.

The early distinction between fat solubility and water solubility still has some relevance in our consideration of vitamins because solubility determines certain characteristics of the way vitamins are absorbed and excreted.

Solubility and toxicity

Water-soluble vitamins, C and the B-complex, are easily absorbed and readily dissolved in urine, a water solution, to be excreted. This ease of excretion means that only small amounts of B vitamins and vitamin C can be stored. Water-soluble vitamins in excess of what is needed are eliminated from the body in the urine and, in general, do not cause problems. As with any generalization, there are exceptions. A recent report described weakness and loss of feeling in the hands, arms, and legs of people who took megadoses of vitamin B6. Illness due to excess of water-soluble vitamins occurs infrequently, but the fact that it does happen suggests the need for prudence in dosing with vitamins.

The fat-soluble vitamins, A, D, E, and K, pose a different problem. First of all, they need the presence of some fat to be absorbed. That is easily accomplished because they are found to be associated with fat in foods. Of greater significance is the fact that they cannot be excreted in the urine so that, once absorbed, they are stored in the body. As a result of this virtually unlimited storage, fat-soluble vitamins have a greater potential for causing toxicity. The levels of these vitamins found in almost all foods are quite safe. (Polar bear liver is an exception but it hardly constitutes a significant part of anyone's diet!) Serious problems can develop, however, from overgenerous use of vitamin supplements. Doses of ten times the recommended intake of vitamin A, or only four to five times the recommended level of vitamin D will, in time, cause severe problems. These amounts may sound unrealistically high, but people have been known to take them with untoward results. Well-meaning parents sometimes give "extra" vitamins to babies and children and end up making them sick instead of healthier. It's the old story that "just because a little is good doesn't mean that more is better."

There is another interesting phenomenon related to vitamin A. Carotene, the yellow-orange pigment that gives carrots their color and is found in all deep yellow and dark green fruits and vegetables, is converted in the body to vitamin A. People who eat very large amounts of these foods, such as a pound of carrots each day, store the carotene and eventually find their skin turning the same yellow-orange. It is not a serious health problem, since the excess carotene is not converted to vitamin A, but it does look strange. When the person stops eating sources of carotene, the color gradually fades away.

The situation with vitamins K and E is a bit different. Vitamin K is rarely taken except for particular medical needs related to its role in blood clotting, and then the levels are carefully controlled. Vitamin E is presently being touted and taken to prevent or cure a whole host of ills. There is no good evidence that it is effective in delaying aging, improving sexual potency, preventing heart disease, or curing anything other than vitamin E deficiency, which is very rare. (It has been suggested that vitamin E is effective in relieving menopausal hot flashes and symptoms of premenstrual tension, and some women report that they find it helpful here. These reports are difficult to evaluate since they deal with symptoms which are hard to measure, and which have been shown to respond to placebos—inactive substances which look, taste, and smell the same as drugs or other substances being tested. More research on the subject is needed.) Fortunately vitamin E does not appear to share the high potential for toxicity of vitamins A and D. With all of its popularity, reports of vitamin E toxicity are as rare as proof of its working miracles.

The functions of vitamins

The specific functions of each vitamin are listed in Table 4:1. Broadly stated, vitamins are essential for all body processes: growth, reproduction, metabolism, and the function of all organ systems. Vitamins achieve these feats in two general ways. Some vitamins serve as regulators of important processes. Vitamin D, for example, helps to control the absorption and metabolism of calcium. It is a key part of the system that regulates the amount of calcium circulating in the blood and stored in the bones. The B vitamins act as coenzymes, nonprotein factors which enzymes must have in order to be effective in metabolism. For instance, pyridoxine, vitamin B6, is needed for the conversion of essential amino acids into the non-essentials. Without pyridoxine it would be impossible to make any amino acids in the body, and they would all have to be obtained from the diet.

Vitamin requirements

The very definition of vitamins indicates that the amounts needed are small. Vitamin requirements are measured in milligrams (one-thousandth of a gram) and micrograms (one-thou-

Table 4:1. The Functions of Vitamins

Vitamin	Function(s)	Effect of Deficiency/excess	Sources
A Retinol	maintains integrity of skin and membranes; ability to see in dim light	loss of ability to see in dim light, itchy, scaly skin blindness; excess: headache, pain in the bones, vomiting; note: hypercarotenemia, due to excess of carotene, a yellow-orange pigment which is converted in the body to vitamin A, causes a yellow-orange discoloration of the skin but no systemic effects	organ meats, egg yolk, butter, cream, fortified milk, margarine, carotene in dark green and deep yellow vegetables and fruits
D Calciferol	absorption and metabolism of calcium	failure to absorb and utilize calcium, leads to rickets, a bone deformity in children, and osteomalacia, a similar disorder in adults; excess: headache, vomiting, deposits of calcium in soft tissues such as heart, blood vessels, and kidneys	formed in skin when exposed to ultraviolet light—this is generally sufficient to meet adult needs; fortified milk, margarine, fish liver oils
E Tocopherol	protects membranes from damage by oxidation	deficiency not seen in healthy people	vegetable oils, whole grains, wheat germ, liver, legumes, fruits and vegetables
K Menadione	blood clotting	deficiency not seen in healthy people	made in adequate amounts by bacteria normally present in the intestine

Vitamins 29

C Ascorbic Acid	needed for "intracellular cement," the substance which holds tissues together formation of collagen iron absorption involved in body's response to stress and infection	scurvy: bleeding gums, loosened teeth, easy bruising, pain in joints poor wound healing	citrus fruits, tomatoes, cabbage, potatoes, melons, berries, peppers, other fruits and vegetables
B1 Thiamin	cofactor for enzymes that metabolize carbohydrate maintain normal function of intestine possibly involved in nerve transmission	beri-beri: depression, irritability, confusion, weakness, loss of appetite damage to heart muscle and brain	liver, meats enriched and whole grains, legumes, nuts
B2 Riboflavin	cofactor in enzyme reactions to release energy from food	redness and cracking of lips, sore tongue	milk, dairy products, enriched grains, organ meats, leafy vegetables
B3 Niacin	cofactor in enzyme reactions to metabolize carbohydrate and fat and to release energy from food	pellagra: skin rash, mental changes, diarrhea excess: large doses cause flushing, itching, burning of skin	meat, fish, eggs, legumes, nuts, milk
B6 Pyridoxine	cofactor for enzyme reactions of proteins and amino acids formation of hemoglobin normal function of nerve tissue	redness, cracking of lips, itchy, scaly skin convulsions in infants excess: weakness, loss of feeling in hands, arms, and legs	organ meats, meat, eggs, yeast, grains, fruits and vegetables
Folic acid Folacin	cofactor for enzyme reactions of proteins, amino acids, and DNA formation of red blood cells	anemia	leafy green vegetables, organ meats, legumes, nuts, milk

Table 4:1. (Continued)

Vitamin	Function(s)	Effect of Deficiency/excess	Sources
B12 Cobalamin	cofactor for enzyme reactions of protein and DNA formation of red blood cells normal function of nerve tissue	dietary deficiency only in strict vegetarians (vegans) pernicious anemia, due to inability to absorb B12	all animal products
Biotin	Cofactor for enzyme reactions of proteins, fats, and carbohydrates	deficiency not seen in healthy people (Biotin can be inactivated by avidin, a substance found in raw, but not cooked, egg white. Very large amounts are needed to have any effect.)	all plant and animal foods made by bacteria normally present in the intestine
Pantothenic Acid	cofactor in enzyme reactions of proteins, fats, and carbohydrates and release of energy	deficiency not seen in healthy people	all plant and animal foods

sandth of a milligram), quantities clearly unrelated to their importance.

It is difficult to determine the minimum amount of a vitamin we need to maintain good health. Many experiments have been done and there is information on the levels of nutrients required under the conditions that were studied, but this knowledge is not easily translated into practical guidance. There are variations from one individual to another, and the requirement for some vitamins is influenced by other components of the diet. In order to be useful, recommendations must allow for these differences and establish levels that apply to the population as a whole. This is exactly the objective of the Food and Nutrition Board of the National Research Council in determining the Recommended Dietary Allowances, better known as the RDA. The RDAs represent the best assessment by a panel of distinguished nutritionists of the amounts of nutrients which should be consumed by healthy Americans. At roughly 5-year intervals, a panel reviews the scientific literature and updates the recommendations according to the best available data. They consider what is known about minimal requirements, age and individual differences, availability of the nutrient from food sources and utilization in the body. For most nutrients, recommendations are set on the high side to allow a margin of safety. While not perfect, the RDAs are the best guidelines we have, and are the most widely used nutritional standards in the United States.

Vitamin deficiencies

What happens when a person consumes too little of a vitamin? In the first stage of a vitamin deficiency, any of the vitamin which has previously been saved is used. Function is maintained but the body's stores are depleted. Once the reserve is gone, the function for which the vitamin is needed begins to decline. If, for example, the vitamin functions as an enzyme cofactor, that enzyme reaction no longer works as well. At this point a careful laboratory analysis will reveal the deficiency although there are no overt signs of it. As the depletion progresses, its effects become more evident until there is a frank, or clinical, deficiency marked by diminished function and changes in physical and/or mental status.

The term "subclinical deficiency" refers to the early stages, when there is biochemical but not clinical evidence of the disorder. The term has also been popularized by those whose motive is the sale of vitamin supplements, thus suggesting that subclinical deficiencies are widespread. Since by definition you can't recognize a subclinical deficiency, this argument suggests that the only recourse is to take supplements to protect yourself. In fact, *there is no evidence of widespread vitamin deficiencies in the United States.* There are individuals, particularly members of low income groups or people who limit their food consumption, whose vitamin intakes are lower than is desirable, but they are not in the majority of the population. All of the necessary vitamins can be obtained from a good mixed diet. The human race survived on food for eons before vitamin supplements hit the market! The woman who is concerned that her diet, or her family's, is inadequate has several choices. One approach, the one I favor, is to improve the diet. If for some reason, or at a particular time, she feels that taking a supplement would also be a good thing to do, then she would be wise to check the label and stay with preparations that contain from half to the full RDA, but no more. This would provide the insurance she may be seeking without the risk of creating imbalances or toxic reactions.

Vitamins and disease prevention

In addition to their established roles in nutrition, vitamins have recently been in the news for their possible role in preventing diseases which have previously been considered nonnutritional. The first excitement came in 1970 when vitamin C was proposed as a preventive and cure for the common cold—the response to this ranged from wild enthusiasm to skepticism to downright disbelief. Many people began popping vitamin C and some scientists began doing serious research. Several years and many experiments later, it appears that megadoses of vitamin C (one to two grams rather than the RDA of 60 milligrams) may somewhat reduce the symptoms and duration of some colds. Studied under controlled conditions, the effect is small. Fortunately, the risk of high levels of vitamin C also appears small; only a few cases of anything more serious than intestinal disturbance have been reported.

The more serious disease to be studied in relation to vitamin intake is cancer. Research in this area is still in its early stages, but it does suggest some safe measures which may be taken.

Surveys have shown that people who consume generous amounts of foods containing vitamin A and carotene, a plant pigment which is converted in the body to vitamin A, have lower rates of several kinds of cancer. It is not clear whether the apparent protection comes from the carotene, the vitamin A itself, or some unidentified factor in the same foods. The data on vitamin C and cancer are even scantier than with vitamin A, but some studies suggest that it, too, may be protective. Based on these observations, a committee of the National Research Council has recommended frequent consumption of foods which are sources of vitamins A and C: citrus fruits, dark green and deep yellow vegetables, and vegetables in the cabbage family. It is important to note that the committee specified that its recommendation applies only to foods and *not to supplements* of individual nutrients, which can be toxic in large amounts.

5
MINERALS

Minerals are defined as inorganic chemical elements. To the chemist, organic chemicals are compounds, found principally in plants and animals, that share certain characteristics. One of these characteristics is their combustibility. When plant or animal matter is burned, all of the organic part is destroyed, leaving only ash which represents the inorganic portion. In the case of humans, the ash is about four per cent of the body weight. Three-fourths of it is composed of calcium and phosphorus, the predominant minerals in the skeleton. The remainder includes iron, sodium, potassium, copper, magnesium, zinc, chromium, and a number of other elements in very small but essential quantities.

Our knowledge of mineral metabolism and requirements is one of the most rapidly expanding areas in nutrition. Because the concentration of most minerals in the body is so low, extensive nutrition research had to await the development of highly sophisticated instruments and techniques. These are now available, enabling scientists to measure and study inorganic components of the body and enlarge the list of those known to play essential metabolic roles.

The functions of minerals

If we were to rank the functions of minerals according to the quantities involved, first place would clearly go to the structural role of *calcium* and *phosphorus*, which make bones and teeth hard and sturdy. Both of these hard tissues begin with a protein matrix that defines the size and shape of the bone or tooth. Calcium and phosphorus are then deposited in the protein to give strength and hardness to the structure.

Minerals also act as cofactors for enzymes in many important reactions ranging from releasing energy from food to copying DNA to make new cells. They serve as regulators of processes as diverse as muscle contraction, blood clotting and the transmission of messages along nerves. Minerals control the amount of water retained within cells and between them. This is another finely tuned mechanism, with sodium and potassium being the most important elements here.

Minerals are important, too, as transporters within the body. The best example of this function is iron which plays a crucial role in carrying oxygen from the lungs to every cell and carbon dioxide from the cells back to the lungs.

Mineral requirements

The quantities of minerals required each day vary from calcium, which can be measured in grams, to iodine, which is measured in micrograms. The six required in the largest amounts are calcium, phosphorus and magnesium, sodium, potassium, and chlorine. Those remaining are often called *trace minerals*, a name that goes back to the days when minute quantities could not be measured accurately, and it was said that only "traces" of them were required.

The minerals listed in Table 5:1 are those for which a function is known and recommended allowances or ranges have been established. For the first six, calcium, phosphorus, magnesium, iron, zinc, and iodine, specific RDAs have been set. The others are known to be essential, but there is not enough information available to determine a recommended level of intake. For these, a "safe and adequate" range has been suggested. These are provisional recommendations designed to provide enough of the nutrient to meet physiological needs without risk of toxic effects from excesses. With more time and research it will no doubt be possible to establish RDAs for these minerals as well. In addition to all of the minerals listed, elements such as mercury, lead, and gold are found in human beings but have no known function. It may be that they are simply deposited in the body as a result of their presence in the environment; perhaps, in time it will be found that they, too, have roles to play.

Mineral deficiencies

Typical American diets are sometimes low in certain of the essential minerals. Inadequate *iron* is the deficiency found most often in this country. Iron is also the one nutrient which women need in larger amounts than men do. Both sexes need to replenish the iron lost as hair grows, skin sloughs off, and cells in the intestines are replaced. Women in their menstruating years have the extra loss of iron in the menstrual flow which must be made up. This averages out, over a month, to one-half to one milligram per day, compared to one milligram per day for all the other losses. In order to maintain iron levels, a woman's RDA for iron is set at 18 milligrams per day to accommodate the daily loss of 1½ to 2 milligrams. This is because of the variability in the absorption of iron from food. Iron from flesh foods, meat, poultry and fish, is well absorbed, but absorption from eggs and vegetable products is less efficient. The presence of meat or vitamin C in a meal enhances the absorption of iron from non-meat sources.

Zinc is another mineral which may be marginal in some U.S. diets. It, too, is absorbed better from animal sources than from vegetables.

Calcium

Many women consume less than the recommended amount of calcium. While calcium occurs in a variety of foods, milk and dairy products are the best sources. Most mothers encourage their children to drink milk but around adolescence, young women often decrease the amount of milk they drink without compensating with other sources of calcium. There is a common notion that once bones and teeth are fully formed, calcium is no longer important. That is not really the case, because calcium is constantly being withdrawn from the bones and a steady supply is needed to replace it. In the teeth, calcium and phosphorus, once deposited, are there to stay. They can be dissolved from the surface (as described in the explanation in Chapter 1 of the role of sugar in dental caries), but are not withdrawn for other use in the body. Bone, on the other hand, acts as a calcium reserve. Rather than just sitting inertly in the bone, the calcium is in a dynamic state, constantly being withdrawn and redeposited. You could compare it to a very active bank account in which a constant balance reflects equal deposits and withdrawals. Calcium,

Table 5:1. Minerals in the Body

Mineral	Function(s)	Effect of Deficiency/excess	Sources
Calcium	structure of bones and teeth nerve transmission muscle contraction blood clotting cardiac function	lack of mineral in bone (also related to Vitamin D)	milk, dairy products, dark green vegetables, seeds, canned salmon and sardines (with bones)
Phosphorus	structure of bones and teeth use of energy in the body	deficiency not seen in healthy people weakness, lack of mineral in bone	protein foods: meat, dairy products, eggs soft drinks
Magnesium	structure of bones and teeth cofactor in enzyme reactions	deficiency rare in healthy people	vegetables, legumes, whole grains
Iron	oxygen transport use of energy	anemia: fatigue, weakness excess: excreted by healthy adults, can be toxic in children	organ meats, meat, dark green vegetables, whole grains, egg yolks
Zinc	cofactor in enzyme reactions	poor growth loss of sense of taste	meat, protein foods, whole grains, legumes
Iodine	in thyroid hormone which regulates many body processes	inadequate amount of thyroid hormone, goiter excess: depressed thyroid function	saltwater fish, food grown in high iodine soils, iodized salt, may be added to bakery products

Minerals 39

Copper	cofactor for release of energy from food, formation of hemoglobin	deficiency (anemia) rarely seen	nuts, seeds, shellfish, organ meats, meat, whole grains, legumes, drinking water
Fluorine	strengthens teeth	caries-susceptible teeth excess: discolored teeth, severe reactions to doses 25× recommended	fluoridated water, tea
Manganese	cofactor in enzyme reactions	deficiency not seen in healthy people	nuts, whole grains, vegetables, fruits
Chromium	normal utilization of carbohydrates	impaired carbohydrate metabolism	animal products, whole grains
Selenium	protects from damage due to oxidation reactions	deficiency not seen in healthy people excess: shown toxic in animals	seafood, organ meats, meat, grains
Molybdenum	cofactor in enzyme reactions	deficiency not seen in healthy people	plant and animal products
Sodium	maintain water balance, nerve transmission, muscle contraction	deficiency only seen during illness or from very profuse sweating; weakness excess: contributes to high blood pressure	salt, salty foods, animal products
Potassium	maintain water balance, nerve transmission, muscle contraction, may help regulate blood pressure	deficiency only seen during illness or from some diuretic drugs	meat, milk, citrus fruits, bananas, melons, potatoes, dark green vegetables, nuts

in addition to its structural role, has several vital regulatory functions and its levels in blood and other tissues must be maintained quite precisely. To accomplish this elegant control, there is a complex system involving vitamin D and hormones produced by the thyroid and parathyroid glands. These regulators determine how efficiently calcium from the diet is absorbed, how much is laid down in and released from bone, and the rate at which it is excreted in urine. Osteoporosis, a gradual loss of mineral from bones, is discussed more fully in Chapter 10, but it should be noted here that women who maintain a liberal calcium intake throughout adulthood are less likely to suffer from the disease than women whose calcium intake is low.

The RDA for calcium for adult women is 800 milligrams (0.8 gram) per day, but some experts advise larger amounts, up to 1.5 grams, to decrease the risk of osteoporosis. The best sources of calcium are dairy products. One cup of milk or yogurt provides 300 milligrams and an ounce of hard cheese has 200. Other foods contain calcium, as listed in Table 5:1, but in smaller amounts. Women who don't consume two or three cups of milk, or its equivalent, each day might well consider supplementing their intake with a calcium preparation.

There are other minerals, most notably *lead* and *mercury*, which find their way from the environment into human beings. These "heavy metals" are highly toxic and have no known metabolic function. Government agencies monitor the food supply to protect the consumer from lead and mercury poisoning. The problem, when it arises, is usually from a non-food source such as old lead-based paint. A few cases have also been reported in women who took bone meal as a dietary supplement. Dolomite, another "natural" source of calcium, may also be contaminated with heavy metals, so if you decide to augment your calcium intake, be careful to use a pure, safe source.

Minerals in foods

The mineral content of grains, fruits and vegetables may vary according to the soil and water in the area where the crops are grown. (This is different from vitamins which are made by the plants and are not dependent on the environment.) The levels in animal products are more consistent, since animals regulate the amounts in their bodies. Pure fats and sugars contain no mineral nutrients.

Whole grains are a good source of several minerals. In the process of refining, however, much of the mineral content is lost. Iron is replaced in enriched flour and other cereal products, but trace elements such as zinc and magnesium generally are not, so that enriched grain products, while nutritious, are not entirely equivalent to whole grain.

Sodium and blood pressure

The mineral sodium is another of those nutrients of which we need a certain amount—but too much can cause a problem. The Food and Nutrition Board has estimated a range of 1100 to 3300 milligrams (1.1 to 3.3 grams) to be safe and adequate, but typical American diets may contain as much as 10 to 15 grams of sodium. Sodium is found in varying amounts in nearly all foods. Animal products generally have the highest levels of naturally occurring sodium. Fruits, grains and legumes are low while vegetables vary widely in their sodium content. The major source of sodium in our diets, however, is ordinary table salt and foods to which salt or other sodium compounds have been added. In fact, salt is so important a source of sodium that some people confuse the two terms. Sodium is a mineral which combines chemically with chlorine to form the compound, sodium chloride, which we refer to as salt. Salt is 40 per cent sodium; one teaspoon contains 2000 milligrams of it.

Hypertension. The concern with dietary sodium arises from its relationship to hypertension, high blood pressure. Research has shown that individuals who habitually consume large amounts of sodium, above the recommended range, run a greater risk of developing high blood pressure than do those who have a more moderate sodium intake. This has led to recommendations that Americans decrease their consumption of salt and salty foods. This recommendation has generated some debate because not everyone who eats a lot of salt becomes hypertensive. Many people, up to 80 per cent of the population, maintain normal blood pressure regardless of what they eat. This has led some scientists to conclude that the general public need not change its use of salt. The problem, though, is that there is no way to distinguish in advance between those who are and those who are not going to develop hypertension. Again, each individual has to make her own decision. In a way, it's a matter of how you want to play the odds. You can eat a high sodium diet and wait to see whether you are one of those who will or will not develop hypertension, or you can limit your sodium to decrease the risk.

Women who wish to decrease their sodium intake can begin with the salt shaker. For most Americans, just using less salt in cooking and not adding more at the table is a good first step. The next is to limit the amounts eaten of salty items such as potato chips and salty crackers and snacks, cured meats, processed cheeses, and salty prepared foods. Special "salt-free" and low-sodium products are on the market but are intended for special, very low-sodium diets and are not needed by well women who simply want to eat in a health-promoting way. Labeling foods with their sodium content remains optional, but more and more food manufacturers are choosing to provide this information, allowing consumers to make more informed food choices.

Selenium

Another mineral worth a special note is selenium. It is a recent addition to the list of essential nutrients. The 1980 edition of the Recommended Dietary Allowances was the first to include it. Animal deficiencies of selenium have been observed and it is known to be a cofactor in certain enzyme systems in humans, so it is considered necessary (although a deficiency in humans has not yet been reported). Preliminary research suggests that low selenium levels might be related to increased risk of some cancers, but this is an area that needs more investigation. Also important is the fact that selenium in excess is highly toxic; the range between the desirable and toxic levels is narrower for selenium than for other mineral nutrients. This means that the selenium in a good mixed diet is essential, but that any addition of selenium to food or supplements must be done very cautiously until we know more about its metabolic properties.

Fluorine

Fluorine, or *fluoride* as it is called in its chemically combined form, plays a valuable role in protecting the teeth from decay. If adequate fluoride is available during the period of tooth formation, it is incorporated into the mineral composition of the teeth, making them harder and more resistant to the damage caused by acid on the tooth surface. Fluoride content of foods may vary according to what is in the environment, but there is no reliable, practical food source of the mineral. For that reason, public health and dental authorities advocate the addition of fluoride to water supplies to afford its protection to all children. In some communities, fluoridation has become a highly controversial political issue despite the fact that when properly employed, fluoridation is a proven safe and effective decay preventive measure.

6
WATER

Water's weight often makes it the scapegoat for an extra five pounds that appear on the scale or for a pair of pants that are suddenly too tight! Although women often think of it in this negative way, water is actually an essential nutrient. Depending on age and fatness, water makes up half to three-fourths of the body; the need for it is second only to the need for oxygen. The length of time that one can survive without water is measured in days, compared to minutes without oxygen and weeks or months without food.

Water's functions

Water's functions include serving as the solvent in which essential substances are absorbed and secreted into, transported around, and excreted from the body. It helps to regulate body temperature by transporting heat and by cooling the body through perspiration. Water lubricates the joints and, in saliva, aids in chewing and swallowing food. And throughout the body, water is a structural element of every tissue and every cell.

Water requirements

The need for water is related to the amount lost each day in urine and feces, in perspiration, and from the lungs as we breathe. Under ordinary circumstances, these add up to two to three quarts per day. Profuse sweating, whether due to high temperatures, strenuous physical activity, or a combination can raise that amount to two to three gallons.

Replacing the water which is lost can be accomplished in a variety of easy ways. The most obvious is through drinking plain water or any beverage which appeals to you. Foods, too, are a source of water. Even dry foods contain some (bread is 35 per cent water), but fruits and vegetables which range from 70 to 95 per cent water are more useful in this respect. The point is that while water is necessary, it can come straight from the tap, in milk, tea, coffee or juices, in soup or pudding, or from an orange or tomato.

Thirst is usually a good indicator of the need for water. The experience of being thirsty during hot weather or after intense exercise is a familiar one. Sometimes, though, special attention must be paid to getting enough water. During heavy exercise, for example, thirst may not keep up with increased fluid needs so that athletes need to remember to take a drink at intervals during training or competition. Older people, too, may not get sufficient water if they rely on thirst alone and should be sure to include six to eight glasses of water, or the equivalent, each day.

PART 2
Women Through the Life Cycle

7
THE ADOLESCENT WOMAN

Adolescence, the period of growing into adulthood, is a time of great change and development, both physical and psychological. All of these processes have an impact on nutrition, too, affecting both nutrient needs and eating patterns.

Growth and nutritional needs

The rate at which people grow changes with age. Growth is rapid in infancy and early childhood and then slows down considerably during the later childhood years. As puberty, the attainment of sexual maturity, approaches, the rate speeds up again to produce an adolescent growth spurt. For a girl, the growth spurt usually begins when she is between ten and twelve years old, about two years before she begins to menstruate. She gains weight and grows taller. This is the time in life when differences in body composition between males and females first appear. Girls lay down proportionally less muscle and more fat than boys, producing the curves of a feminine figure. Bone mineralization, the deposition of calcium and phosphorus in the bones, takes place in both sexes, with boys developing heavier skeletons than girls. Maturation comes several years later for boys than for girls, in whom these processes are completed about three or four years after menstruation has begun, or at about 16 to 18 years of age.

This increase in physical growth is reflected in the adolescent's increased nutritional needs. The RDAs for all nutrients are at their maximum (except for the special needs of pregnancy) between the ages of 11 and 18. Girls' need for energy is estimated to be at its highest at 11 to 14 years old. In later adolescence, energy needed for growth is still high but the increase is commonly offset by a decrease in physical activity. The RDAs for protein, certain B vitamins (thiamin, riboflavin, and niacin) and vitamin D also peak during adolescence and then decrease. Other vitamin needs stay at the same level through adulthood. With the beginning of menstruation, the requirement for iron increases and stays elevated until menopause. The RDAs for the remaining minerals hold constant in adolescence and adulthood.

Adolescent eating patterns

During the very time that the growth spurt is increasing the body's demand for all nutrients, other facets of adolescence often lead to changes in eating habits. As the adolescent girl grows into womanhood, she is defining herself and establishing her own independent identity. Her friends become more important in her life and her family less influential. Her ideas about how she should look and what and when she should eat may also change.

The adolescent assumes more responsibility for her own health and nutrition as eating with friends often replaces some of the meals and snacks which used to be eaten at home. Snacks may become a problem now, adding more calories than nutrients to the day's intake. There is nothing wrong with eating some foods just for fun, but the wise young woman will choose good, nutritious foods for most of her snacks. The possibilities include fresh fruits and vegetables and juices, cheese and whole grain crackers, pretzels, yogurt, or a "trail mix" combination of dried fruit and nuts. Ice cream, milkshakes, nuts, and pizza are also good food although they are higher in calories, plus salt in the pizza. And there is nothing wrong with eating leftover "real food" as a snack. Sweets, chips and other fat, salty snacks, sodas and the like are best kept in the "occasional" rather than the "regular" category.

Physical appearance is especially important to adolescents, and girls are often dissatisfied with their figures. Reasonable concern about weight can be a good thing. Since overweight adolescents are likely to become overweight adults, this is a good time to establish patterns of eating and physical activity which will promote long-term health and fitness.

On the other hand, excessive concern or unrealistic standards of thinness can pose a problem. Many adolescents try to lose weight by going on fad diets or staging "crash programs," severely restricting both the amount and kinds of foods they eat. The fact that young women use these approaches repeatedly shows that, in the long run, they don't work. And if done too frequently or for more than a few days, extreme diets are dangerous. It is far healthier, and more effective, to eat sanely and exercise regularly to maintain weight and fitness. Estimated calorie needs for adolescents range from 1200 to 3000 per day. At levels below 1000 calories per day, it is impossible for a young woman to meet her vitamin and mineral requirements, so this should be considered a minimum for extended use. Increasing physical activity, rather than decreasing food intake below this level, will be effective in enhancing efforts at weight control and maintaining good health and fitness.

Realistically, there will probably always be times when an adolescent will want to shed a few pounds in a big hurry, perhaps to look her best for a special event. This is one time when it would be appropriate to use a multivitamin supplement. It is important to realize that no matter what the incentive to reduce, cutting calories below 600 per day is dangerous and ought not be done. (See Chapter 12 for specific suggestions on weight control.)

Anorexia nervosa

Occasionally an adolescent or young woman finds that her weight loss efforts get out of control. She may start out just trying to lose a few pounds, then a few more and a few more and rather than stop her diet when she reaches a good weight, she continues to diet and lose more weight. She still thinks she is too heavy when to the rest of the world, she looks very thin. This problem, called anorexia nervosa, can be serious and dangerous. The severe malnutrition can cause a young woman's hair and skin to change, her menstrual periods to stop, and eventually it threatens her life. Anorexia nervosa is not something a young woman can control by herself; correcting it requires understanding and skillful treatment. Anyone who suffers from this problem should get professional help promptly.

Acne

Acne is another problem which plagues adolescents, affecting from 85 to 100 per cent of teenagers to some degree. Many popular beliefs and recommendations concerning the cause and treatment of acne involve diet. Chocolate, sweets, cola and other soft drinks, and fried or fatty foods are often cited as items which cause acne; it is often claimed that they should be eliminated from the diet. In fact, there is no scientific evidence that eating or drinking any of these products affects acne. Large amounts of alcohol do aggravate acne, as does iodine in the quantities found in some medications such as cough syrups. The amounts of iodine in foods are generally not a problem. If an individual notices that something she eats or drinks does lead to her skin breaking out, she should avoid that item, but there is no need for every adolescent with acne, which means nearly every adolescent, to restrict her diet.

A good diet, however, can help to keep skin healthy and clear. Research has shown that people with severe acne tend to eat diets which are low in zinc, vitamin A, and unsaturated fat, nutrients which can be supplied by a balanced diet.

Vitamin A and compounds chemically related to it are also used in the treatment of acne. At these times, the vitamin and its analogs are acting as drugs and must be respected as such. Because of its toxicity, vitamin A therapy needs careful medical supervision and should never be used as a "do it yourself project."

Importance of nutrition in adolescence

Good nutrition during adolescence is critically important, not just to establish good habits for adulthood, but because the young woman's body is maturing and preparing biologically to be able to bear children. Research has shown that the health and nutritional status of women prior to their becoming pregnant has a significant effect on pregnancy. Even the adolescent who considers having a family a very distant part of her life should realize that her physical development during these years will be important to her as an adult.

The pregnant adolescent

When an adolescent who is still completing her own development becomes pregnant, she adds the nutritional needs of pregnancy to her already high requirements. The RDA for protein, for example, is increased from 46 to 76 grams per day. Vitamin A goes from 800 to 1000 micrograms daily, vitamin C from 60 to 80 milligrams, and calcium from 1200 to 1600 milligrams. There are similar increases for the other vitamins and minerals.

Meeting these requirements demands careful planning. Meals and snacks should be composed of good, nutritious foods; there is little room for high calorie, low nutrient items. (Chapter 9 offers more information on nutrition in pregnancy.) Since the young expectant mother has special needs, it is important that she seek medical care early in her pregnancy. At the same time, she can call upon a registered dietitian or nutritionist to help her plan menus that will satisfy her and provide the nutrients she needs for a healthy pregnancy.

Here are some menus to suggest the kind of meals and snacks which would provide good nutrition for adolescents. The menus for the first day provide a total of 1775 calories; for the second day, 1950 calories; and the third day, 2050 calories.

Day 1

Breakfast:
    orange juice, ½ cup
    whole wheat toast, 1 slice
    cheddar cheese, 2 ounces
    hot chocolate, 1 cup

Lunch:
    tomato soup (made with milk), 1 cup
    turkey sandwich on rye bread
    carrot and celery sticks
    peach

Snack:
    graham crackers, 2
    low fat milk, 1 cup

Dinner:
    beef stew (3 ½ ounces lean beef, onions, peas, tomato)
    noodles, ½ cup
    green salad, 1 cup
    baked apple

Snack:
    popcorn, 1 cup
    apple juice, 1 cup

Day 2

Breakfast:
    corn flakes, ⅔ cup
    strawberries, ½ cup
    low fat milk, ½ cup
    hot chocolate, 1 cup

Lunch:
    grilled cheese sandwich
    low fat milk, 1 cup
    fresh orange

Snack:
    pretzels, 2 ounces
    milkshake, 1 cup

Dinner:
    roast chicken, 3 ½ ounces
    brown rice, ½ cup
    broccoli, 1 large stalk
    sliced tomato salad
    1 roll with 1 teaspoon butter or margarine
    chocolate cake, 1 slice

Snack:
    banana

Day 3

Breakfast:
    orange juice, ½ cup
    French toast, 2 slices, with maple syrup or jam
    hot chocolate, 1 cup

Lunch:
    hamburger, on roll, with lettuce and tomato
    low fat milk, 1 cup

Snack:
    cheese pizza, 1 slice
    soft drink, 1 cup

Dinner:
    baked fish, 3 ½ ounces
    baked potato, 1 medium, with 2 tablespoons yogurt
    peas, ½ cup
    cucumber salad, ½ cup
    butterscotch pudding, ½ cup

Snack:
    raisins, 1 ounce
    peanuts, 1 ounce
    low fat milk, 1 cup

8
THE ADULT WOMAN

After the growth and development of the adolescent years are completed, the adult woman enters a more stable time of life. Nutritional needs decline from the high levels of adolescence and remain fairly constant. The only major nutritional adjustments during these years are for pregnancy and breastfeeding and for changes in levels of physical activity. (These will be discussed in Chapters 9 and 12). This doesn't mean, though, that good nutrition is any less important during adulthood. The demanding schedule of today's woman requires her to stay in top condition. Eating wisely and exercising regularly will go a long way towards maintaining good health and vigor throughout the adult years.

Part I of this book described the nutrients and gave some suggestions about wise food choices and Part IV has more information on food selection and meal planning. This chapter focuses on the particular needs and concerns of women between adolescence and menopause.

Iron

Of all the nutrients, the one most likely to be low in the diets of adult women is iron. The young woman's need for this mineral increased by 50 per cent when she began to menstruate; it remains at that level until her menstruation ceases. To meet this need, women should include good sources of iron in their diets each day. Iron in meat, poultry and fish is absorbed more efficiently than iron in eggs, grains, legumes, and dark green vegetables. To increase the absorption of iron from these other good sources, include a few ounces of meat or a fruit or vegetable which is rich in vitamin C in the meal. Another strategy to increase the iron in the diet is to use old-fashioned cast-iron cookware. Cooking in cast iron dissolves small amounts of iron from the pot and adds it to the food.

We should note here that the RDA for iron for adolescent and adult women has been set at 18 milligrams per day, an amount few women consume. In fact, it is virtually impossible for most women to get 18 milligrams of iron regularly. To do so would require either eating unrealistic amounts of high-iron foods or pushing the total calorie level much too high. Does this mean that iron supplements are a must? Not necessarily. It is possible that the RDA, in its objective of establishing an adequate level for nearly all women, overestimates the iron requirement of many or most women. Moreover, the RDA is based on certain cautious assumptions about how iron in the diet is used by the body. A woman who is in need of iron might use what is in her food more efficiently than is assumed. Supplementation, then, is an individual matter, best based on the state of each woman's iron nutrition. For a healthy woman who eats a good diet, supplements are probably unnecessary but safe to take in reasonable amounts (equal to the RDA.) One caution, though, is important. If there are small children in the household, iron supplements, like all medications, should be stored safely out of reach. Although problems of toxicity are rarely encountered in healthy adults, each year about 2000 American children require treatment for iron poisoning, usually from helping themselves to their parents' supplements.

Calcium and bone health

The effects of low levels of calcium are not as detectable as are low levels of iron during the years when a woman is menstruating, but the amount of calcium a woman consumes during her middle years can make a significant difference later on. The importance of calcium lies in the value of a liberal intake before menopause to lessen the risk of osteoporosis afterwards. *Osteoporosis*, a decrease in the amount of bone which often leads to decreased stature and bone fractures, becomes a serious problem for women in the post-menopausal years. (See Chapter 10 for a more complete discussion of osteoporosis.) Its cause and treatment involve more complex mechanisms than merely the amount of calcium in the diet; however, research has shown that women who have maintained a good calcium intake over the years are less likely to suffer from osteoporosis than are women who have consumed low calcium diets. Unfortunately, women tend to cut down on calcium-rich dairy products in order to cut calories, so that the amount of calcium is often low in women's diets.

The RDA for calcium for adult women is 800 milligrams per day; some experts feel that a larger amount, 1000 to 1200 milligrams, affords better protection from osteoporosis. (The average woman's diet has 400 to 500 milligrams of calcium daily.) To put those amounts in the context of food, a cup of milk provides about 300 milligrams of calcium, a half-cup serving of a dark green vegetable has 175 milligrams (except for spinach and beet greens in which the calcium is in a form which is not well absorbed), three ounces of canned salmon or sardines (with bones) has 250-350 milligrams, a one-cup serving of legumes averages 200 milligrams, and most other foods are considerably lower. Nuts, especially almonds, and seeds, such as sesame and sunflower, are also good sources of calcium, but few people eat them in quantities large enough to be important sources of calcium in the diet.

Certainly every bit helps, and the calcium in green vegetables, legumes, and other foods can add up to a substantial amount. But it is clear from the figures that it is difficult to achieve a generous calcium intake without dairy products. There are a variety of ways to include milk in the diet. The most obvious is to drink a couple of glasses of milk, preferably skim or low fat, each day. Other possibilities include using the milk in soups and desserts or substituting yogurt or cheese. Yogurt has the same nutritional value as the milk from which it is made. Cheese has less water in it so that 1½ ounces of a hard cheese such as cheddar or Swiss has the same amount of calcium as one cup of milk. (Cheese also has a higher fat content so the woman who depends on it for her calcium might want to cut down on other sources of fat.) Cottage cheese and cream cheese are lower in calcium than the hard cheeses. To get the equivalent of one cup of milk requires one and a half cups of cottage cheese or 13 ounces of cream cheese. A handy product for increasing calcium intake is skim milk powder. It can be added to liquid milk or other foods to increase their calcium value.

Calcium supplements

As with other nutrients, calcium is best obtained from a good diet. The foods provide other minerals and vitamins and in the case of milk, lactose aids in utilization of the calcium. Many women, however, are unable to reach the desired level of 1000 to 1200 milligrams of calcium each day. They may have a low tolerance for dairy products or find it impractical to include an average of three servings each day. These women might well consider taking extra calcium to supplement their diets. There are several different calcium preparations on the market today. In each of them calcium is combined with some other chemicals to form a calcium compound; when reading the label, you should look for the amount of elemental calcium, not the total weight of the compound, in each tablet. Supplements prepared from calcium carbonate have the advantages of having the highest per cent of elemental calcium and of being well absorbed.

One reasonable approach is to estimate your usual calcium intake, using the values given above for high calcium foods, and supplement that to bring your total up to 1000 to 1200 milligrams. Of course, any individual questions or concerns should be discussed with a physician, nurse or registered dietitian.

Exercise

Eating enough calcium is only part of what it takes to keep bones healthy; exercise also plays a role. Physical activity affects the balance between calcium being deposited in and withdrawn from the bones: the active woman will use her supply of calcium to better advantage than the sedentary woman will. The exercise does not have to be intense; it does have to be regular. The best form of exercise is one that is enjoyable as well as practical so that it can become part of the daily routine. Running, bicycling and brisk walking are just some of the possibilities.

Premenstrual syndrome

Premenstrual syndrome is a problem which has been well publicized but remains poorly understood. The term describes a cluster of symptoms which many women experience several days before their menstrual periods begin. Symptoms of PMS include swelling and tenderness of the breasts, a feeling of abdominal bloating, swelling of hands and feet, headache, fatigue and depression or irritability and tension, increased appetite and thirst, food cravings, skin eruptions and constipation. The symptoms may vary from month to month and from woman to woman.

For some women the symptoms are minor and can easily be ignored. Others are more severely affected and find their lives disrupted for days each month. Researchers are trying to unravel the cause of PMS: there is no evidence that it is a nutritional disease but dietary measures often relieve the symptoms, and for many women are all the treatment they need.

The changes in the diet which are recommended for the woman with PMS are related directly to her symptoms. Since fluid retention is part of the problem, the first step is to decrease *salt* intake. That means avoiding both the salt shaker and salty foods, a task which can be difficult for the woman who finds herself craving salt. There really isn't any easy answer for her, just will power, determination, and concentration on the benefit to be gained from the abstinence. It may also help to know that the first few weeks of a low-salt diet are the hardest. After several weeks of not adding salt to food, the palate adjusts to the change and food tastes just as good as it used to when salt was added to it.

Caffeine also goes on the "avoid" list for the woman with PMS. It is hardly more than common sense to stay away from a stimulant when irritability and tension are the problems. Good-tasting decaffeinated coffees and teas make this measure an easy one to live with, although the woman who has been in the habit of drinking large amounts of coffee or tea may miss the stimulating effects of caffeine at first. Again, perseverance through the period of adjustment will pay off in feeling better later.

After cutting salt and caffeine comes a more comprehensive *change in eating habits*. Premenstrual syndrome is not the same thing as hypoglycemia, low blood sugar, but the type of diet used to treat hypoglycemia frequently relieves the symptoms of PMS. There are two main features of this diet: eating five or six times a day—and reducing the intake of simple carbohydrates. Meals should be kept on the light side and supplemented with high protein snacks in between. Carbohydrates should be mainly complex, or starches, with moderate amounts of sugars from fruits and milk and little or no refined sugars and sweets. The following is a sample meal pattern.

breakfast:	4 ounces fruit juice
	½ cup cereal
	4 ounces skim or low fat milk
	decaffeinated coffee
mid-morning:	1 ounce cheese
	2 unsalted whole grain crackers
	decaffeinated coffee
lunch:	3 ounces meat, fish, poultry or substitute
	1 slice whole grain bread
	salad or cooked vegetable
	fresh fruit
	decaffeinated tea
mid-afternoon:	2 tablespoons peanut butter
	1 slice whole grain bread
	8 ounces skim or low fat milk
dinner:	soup
	3 ounces meat or substitute
	½ cup potato, rice, or noodles
	½ cup vegetables
	salad
	fresh fruit
	decaffeinated tea or coffee
bedtime:	½ cup cottage cheese
	2 graham crackers

Following these restrictions and eating patterns is most important shortly before and during the premenstrual period, but it makes sense to adhere to them to a reasonable degree all month. It saves keeping track of the calendar each month to anticipate the symptoms and more important, leads to the new style becoming habitual rather than a repeated, monthly struggle.

Vitamins, particularly E and B6, have been tried and recommended by some as a source of relief for PMS. More research needs to be done to determine how effective these supplements really are. Since very high doses of B6 have proven toxic, a woman who wishes to try using this vitamin should seek medical advice from her physician or a reputable PMS clinic.

Exercise is the final ingredient in an anti-PMS program. Like some of the other recommended measures, exercise may not be directly related to the cause of premenstrual syndrome, but its effect is to reduce feelings of stress and tension and increase a sense of well-being. There are no specific exercises that should be done; running, biking, swimming, or brisk walking, done regularly, contribute both to the relief of PMS and to good health in general.

Contraceptives

Both oral contraceptives and intrauterine contraceptive devices cause changes in a woman's body which can have implications for nutrition.

Oral contraceptives produce a wide variety of metabolic effects involving several vitamins and minerals. The most important are changes in the absorption and use of vitamin B6, folic acid, and vitamin C, so that women taking OCs need to have more of these vitamins. A generous intake of fruits and vegetables is an easy way to get enough of these nutrients.

Contrary to the increased vitamin needs, iron requirements may be lower in women on oral contraceptives due to a decrease in the amount of menstrual flow. Women who use intrauterine contraceptive devices, on the other hand, frequently experience a heavier flow and therefore may need to be more attentive to iron in their diets.

Weight gain may be another side effect of oral contraceptives. To the extent that water retention is part of the problem, cutting salt intake can help. Other than that, the woman who takes OCs can use the same approach of a good diet and sufficient exercise as any woman who is concerned with controlling her weight.

Bulimia and anorexia

In addition to the nutritional concerns related to their special physiology, women are particularly susceptible to developing the extreme patterns of eating known as anorexia nervosa and bulimia or bulimarexia.

Anorexia nervosa usually begins during adolescence but may extend into adulthood. The young woman who has this problem may have begun with a fairly ordinary weight loss program but then fails to recognize that her weight is getting too low. She continues at a high level of physical activity and low level of caloric intake, thinking herself fat while to the rest of the world she appears painfully thin. If unchecked, anorexia nervosa can lead to severe medical problems and even death.

Bulimia, binge eating, or bulimarexia, bingeing and purging, may produce less visible change in the body than anorexia but can also have severe consequences. These disorders, which may be more common in adult women, are marked by the consumption of large amounts of high calorie foods within fairly short periods of time. The woman with bulimia may put away 15,000 to 20,000 calories' worth of ice cream, cookies, cake, or pastries in one sitting. She stops only when her stomach will hold no more, at which time she may induce vomiting to purge herself of the excess. Large doses of laxatives or diuretics may also be used as means of purging. Each of these methods can disrupt normal metabolic processes and cause serious illness. Depending on the balance she strikes between eating and purging, a woman with this disease may be of normal weight or be overweight.

A full discussion of these eating disorders is beyond the scope of this book. It is important, though, to recognize that they occur in women about ten times more often than in men, that they are serious problems that must be treated professionally, and that help is available. Treatment includes medical attention to any metabolic problems, some type of counseling or therapy to resolve the psychological component, and ideally, nutritional counseling to help the woman get back to healthy eating.

9
THE PREGNANT WOMAN AND NURSING MOTHER

Pregnancy is a special time for a woman . . . and for the child she is carrying. You know, when you are pregnant, that you are now responsible for the health of two people and you may be inundated with advice on what to do, what to eat, and what to expect. Friends and relatives regale you with tales of their experiences and recommendations that may—or may not—be appropriate for you and your growing baby. One may remind you that you are "eating for two" while another cautions you against gaining too much weight. Sorting it all out can be difficult! Since much of the advice and many of the myths concern nutrition and diet, this chapter will help you to understand the changing nutritional needs during pregnancy and to find practical ways to meet your needs. The information and suggestions are all general, but it is important to remember that no general recommendations can replace the counsel of a physician or nurse-midwife who knows the woman and the particular circumstances of her pregnancy. Pregnancy is a unique period in a woman's life; good prenatal care will help to ensure the health of the mother and her baby.

Weight gain

Recommendations about weight gain during pregnancy sometimes seem like hemlines, rising and falling apparently inexplicably. Actually, there is an explanation to be found in the evolution of scientists' understanding of pregnancy and how best to promote the health of mother and baby. In the old days, pregnant women commonly gained large amounts of weight. It's not unusual to hear tales of 50 and 60-pound pregnancies! Then, about the time of the first World War, it was thought that some of the complications of pregnancy could be prevented by restricting weight gain. That view prevailed for quite a while and in the '50s and '60s, women were urged to limit their gains to 15 to 20 pounds. More recently, obstetricians have learned that those recommendations were too restrictive and now they take a more liberal view. Current thinking favors a gain in the range of 24 to 28 pounds, with little increase during the first three months and then a slow, steady gain. That range assumes that the woman is at her desirable weight when she becomes pregnant. A woman who is underweight would do well to gain more, roughly 24 to 28 pounds plus what it would take to reach her desirable weight. The overweight woman, on the other hand, should not use pregnancy as a time to try to get down to her desirable weight. She should be careful about her diet, like all pregnant women, but postpone any thought of weight reduction until after the baby is born. The top priority during pregnancy has to be *eating a good diet that provides all of the nutrients needed to make a healthy baby.*

About 20 pounds of the mother's weight gain can be accounted for by the baby and by changes in the mother's body. In an "average" normal pregnancy, this weight is divided (in pounds) like this:

baby	7–7.5
placenta	1–1.5
amniotic fluid	2
growth of uterus	2–2.5
enlargement of breasts	1–3
increased blood	3–4

Remember that these are average ranges, not exact figures for any individual. Each woman will gain in her own way.

The extra weight above 20 pounds is fat which is put down

so that the mother will have some energy in reserve for the busy time after the baby is born. It's a normal part of the body's preparation for birth and breastfeeding. Most women have no difficulty using up 10 pounds or so of this stored energy, so the woman who gains a total of 30 pounds can return easily to her prepregnant weight in two or three months after the baby is born. A women who gains much more than 30 pounds is likely to have more trouble getting back to her usual weight.

One note of caution on the subject of gaining weight: it is normal to retain some fluid during the last three months of pregnancy, but a sudden, rapid weight gain (three pounds or more in a week) may indicate excessive fluid retention; this is cause for a call to the physician or nurse.

Nutrient needs during pregnancy

As you would expect, a pregnant woman's need for all nutrients increases. Early in pregnancy, when the fetus is still tiny, the increases are small. That doesn't mean, though, that good nutrition can wait. Having the right amounts of nutrients is important for the marvelous process by which a single cell turns into a complete human being. And as pregnancy progresses and the baby is fully formed and getting larger, the mother needs more of everything to support the baby's growth and the changes in her own body.

Energy

Pregnancy increases energy requirements in several ways. During pregnancy, a woman's metabolic rate speeds up and it takes more energy, or calories, to maintain her. Second is the more obvious need for extra energy to build new tissue in the mother and her baby. There is another subtle factor involved; it takes more energy to move a larger body. As a woman's weight increases she uses more calories to do any kind of physical activity. Many women, however, are less active during pregnancy and the two changes often balance out. But this shouldn't be taken as advice against being active. On the contrary, physical activity is just as healthful during pregnancy as at any other time, and most women do well to include it in their daily routines. In some areas there are prenatal exercise classes designed especially for pregnant women, should that kind of activity appeal to you. (If in doubt, or if you engage in super-strenuous sports or training, check with your medical adviser for individual guidance.)

It has been estimated that over the nine months of pregnancy, a woman needs an extra 80,000 calories beyond her usual requirements. That looks like quite a lot, doesn't it? It seems more reasonable when you look at it on a daily basis. Since needs are smaller early in pregnancy, an additional 150 calories per day are recommended during the first three months. From the fourth month until the baby is born, the recommendation is to add 350 calories each day. Of course, these are general or average values, not exact numbers for any particular woman. The best criterion for each woman is her weight gain. If she is gaining at a suitable rate, then her calorie intake is fine. If weight is increasing too rapidly or too slowly, then some dietary adjustment is called for.

Protein

By the time a baby is born its body and its mother's have accumulated about two pounds of pure protein. If you were to divide that amount by the length of pregnancy you would get about four grams of protein per day. The RDA for protein is much higher than that, an additional 30 grams above the regular RDA. The recommendation is so high partly because it takes about ten grams of protein in the diet to make four grams of body protein, and partly because a generous protein intake is one factor which leads to a healthy newborn. Since most Americans consume more than the RDA for protein, getting enough during pregnancy poses no problem.

Vitamins and minerals

As you would expect, a woman needs more of all the vitamins during pregnancy. Vitamin A plays a role in the early stages when specific organs are developing from a mass of undifferentiated cells. Many of the B vitamins are used in the metabolic reactions that release energy from food and use it in the body; when more energy is being used, more of these vitamins are necessary. Other B vitamins are involved in the processes that form new cells and build protein from amino acids. Vitamin C, too, is needed to build new tissue. Vitamin D promotes the absorption of calcium and its incorporation into bones and teeth. Each of these processes is part of what happens as an unborn baby grows, so it makes sense that a woman's need for vitamins increases during pregnancy.

In the same way, additional minerals are needed during pregnancy. There is an old saying, "for every child a tooth." That's not true, for the *calcium* in a woman's teeth is unaffected by pregnancy. What is true is that a baby is born with about 30 grams of calcium in its body, calcium that needs to be supplied by the mother's diet. If you do the 30 grams divided by the length of pregnancy arithmetic, you get 100 milligrams per day. But because not all the calcium you eat is absorbed, the RDA for calcium is increased 400 milligrams, a 50 per cent increase.

The pregnant woman's increased need for *iron* is even more striking. In the later part of its prenatal life, a baby stores iron to an extent that it never will again. It's part of the preparation for living on a diet of milk, which is low in iron, during early infancy. Getting enough iron from the diet poses a problem for pregnant women. This becomes quite clear when you consider that most non-pregnant women consume less than the recommended amount of this mineral. Because of this, most experts advise iron supplements during pregnancy. Adding 30 to 60 milligrams per day (and more for women whose iron level is low) has become a routine part of prenatal care.

Sodium is another nutrient which has been the subject of new knowledge and changing recommendations. Pre-eclampsia and eclampsia, serious complications of pregnancy, are marked by fluid retention and elevated blood pressure. Since sodium is involved in both fluid balance and blood pressure regulation, it seemed logical to restrict sodium intake in an effort to prevent these problems; for years pregnant women were counseled to do just that. More recent research has shown that a normal sodium intake does not cause complications of pregnancy and that pregnant women do well by maintaining their usual level of sodium.

Nutrient sources: food and supplements

Good nutrition is so important a part of prenatal care that most women today are advised both to eat well and to take a multivitamin and mineral supplement. As we have noted, even good diets are often below the recommended level of iron. Zinc and folic acid (a B vitamin) also tend to be low compared to the increased requirements of pregnancy. To cover these specific needs and add a measure of insurance, the use of nutrient supplements has become routine.

Remember, though, that supplements are intended to add to—and not replace—a healthy diet. Eating well is a key part of total prenatal care, and no pill contains all of the trace elements, protein, fiber, and other nutrients found in a variety of good food. The basics of meal planning and food choices described in Chapter 15 apply just as well to the pregnant woman. If she starts out with a good diet, she needs only to make some judicious additions: one to two glasses of skim or low fat milk or the equivalent in yogurt, cheese or other dairy products, and an extra serving of a fruit or vegetable. It is also a good idea to drink a few extra glasses of water.

Here is a sample meal pattern showing one way to eat well.

  breakfast: citrus fruit or juice
       whole grain bread or cereal
       milk or substitute
       beverage
  snack: milk or substitute
  lunch: meat or substitute
       whole grain bread or crackers
       vegetables and/or fruit
       milk or substitute
       beverage
  snack: fruit
  dinner: meat or substitute
       starch, such as rice, pasta, or potato
       vegetable
       whole grain bread
       salad
       fruit or dessert
       beverage
  snack: milk or substitute

Translated into food, the pattern might look like this:

  breakfast: orange juice
       whole grain cereal with raisins
       whole wheat toast with butter or margarine
       skim or low fat milk
       coffee or tea

snack: hot chocolate, made with milk
lunch: tuna salad sandwich with lettuce and tomato, on rye bread
small salad
baked custard
decaffeinated coffee or tea
snack: banana
dinner: broiled chicken
baked potato with yogurt
broccoli
dinner roll with butter or margarine
green salad
melon
decaffeinated coffee or tea
snack: skim or low fat milk

Or like this:

breakfast: half grapefruit
whole wheat toast (2 slices) with butter or margarine
cottage cheese
skim or low fat milk
coffee or tea
snack: skim or low fat milk
lunch: split pea soup
cheddar cheese
rye crackers
carrot and celery sticks
decaffeinated tea or coffee
snack: peach
dinner: baked fish
rice
peas with mushrooms
whole wheat roll with butter or margarine
tomato salad
baked apple
decaffeinated coffee or tea
snack: yogurt with fresh fruit

The pattern and menus illustrate one of the many ways to eat healthily. They are intended to give you ideas, not to impose a rigid rule; each woman will devise her own plan to suit her particular needs and preferences. The menus, too, are very basic.

Most women would probably add such extras as dressing on the salad or a cookie with a glass of milk. Some would have additional snacks or a dessert of ice cream, cake or pie. Assuming that weight gain is progressing at a desirable rate, any of these changes would be fine. So would shifting foods from one meal or snack to another. What is important is that by the end of the day the pregnant woman has eaten enough of the basic foods to provide for her nutritional needs.

Items To Avoid

Caffeine

You may have noticed that decaffeinated beverages were specified in most of the sample menus. The reason for this is that questions have been raised about the safety of caffeine during pregnancy. Experiments on animals have shown that high doses of caffeine during pregnancy can cause malformations in the young. There is no good evidence that this happens in humans or that ordinary amounts of caffeine are harmful; nonetheless, it is reasonable to be cautious. Until we know with certainty what effect caffeine has on humans, and in what amounts, common sense suggests that pregnant women not drink large quantities of caffeinated beverages. That means limiting regular tea and coffee, cola and other caffeinated soft drinks, chocolate, and medications which contain caffeine. The menus were written with a compromise, regular tea or coffee at breakfast and decaffeinated beverages for the rest of the day. This seems reasonable for most women. Those who want to play it extra safe can avoid caffeine entirely. Herbal teas enjoy great popularity with many people trying to avoid caffeine. While they are in most cases caffeine-free, little is known about some of the other substances they contain. Moderate consumption—a cup or two—should be all right, but drinking large amounts is probably not a good idea. Wiser choices would include milk, fruit juices, and plain club soda.

Alcohol

The Surgeon General of the United States has issued a warning about the hazards of alcohol consumption during pregnancy. The warning is intended to prevent the birth of babies with fetal alcohol syndrome, a problem which occurs in babies born to mothers who drink heavily. The baby with fetal alcohol syndrome is small, has a recognizably different appearance, may be irritable in its early days, and suffers from mental retardation.

The full effects of fetal alcohol syndrome are seen in babies born to women who frequently drink five ounces or more of alcohol (equivalent to 10 jiggers of whiskey, glasses of wine or bottles of beer) per day. It is quite clear that this amount of alcohol poses a danger, and a woman who is accustomed to drinking it, or more, should seek help in cutting her alcohol intake. What is not clear is the effect of smaller amounts of alcohol. While many women have an occasional cocktail or glass of wine during pregnancy and deliver fine, healthy babies, research has not been able to show a cut-off point. That is, no one can say that below a certain amount, alcohol has no effect on the developing baby. It's another case where common sense dictates prudence. It doesn't mean that a glass of wine on a special occasion will damage the unborn baby, but that in general, non-alcoholic beverages are to be preferred during pregnancy. On this subject, too, a woman who has any concerns should discuss them with her doctor or nurse.

Tobacco

There is no question about the health effects of smoking; it is bad for the mother and the baby. It is not the purpose of this chapter or this book to detail the risks associated with tobacco: they have been highly publicized and are generally known. What we note here is that smokers' blood carries less oxygen than non-smokers' blood, and that women who smoke have smaller babies than women who do not smoke.

It is also true that knowing one more fact about the effects of smoking won't necessarily make it easier to stop! On the other hand, perhaps the realization that she is now responsible for the health of two people will give the expectant mother the extra motivation she needs to kick the smoking habit. Most communities have smoking cessation programs available to offer guidance and moral support to smokers who find it too hard to change by themselves; pregnancy would be a fine time for a woman to take advantage of such a program. Ideally, pregnant women will manage to stop smoking completely, but even those who are unable to can achieve something. Since the effects of smoking are proportional to the number of cigarettes smoked, any decrease is a step in the right direction.

Handling Common Problems

Nausea and vomiting

Early in pregnancy many women experience bouts of nausea that may or may not lead to vomiting. Since the symptoms are often at their worst at the beginning of the day, they are commonly called "morning sickness" (although there are women who think the name should be "morning-afternoon-evening sickness"). The cause of the problem is not completely understood, although it seems to involve the body's hormonal adjustments to being pregnant. "Morning" or "all-day" sickness rarely causes any serious problems and usually subsides after the third month, but until then it can make a woman mightily uncomfortable!

Fortunately, there are some simple measures which usually relieve the worst of the discomfort. First, and most time-honored, is eating plain, dry crackers. If nausea is a problem first thing in the morning, it helps to eat a few crackers before getting out of bed. A box can be kept on the night table or put there in the evening to be ready for the morning.

Changing eating patterns is also helpful. Keeping meals light, and snacking in-between may relieve the nausea, as will avoiding rich and heavy foods. Drinking fluids apart from meals is another useful measure. It is important to maintain fluid intake, but during early pregnancy women may be more comfortable if they have their beverages between meals rather than with them.

These tactics won't eliminate the problem but should help in living with it. Occasionally the nausea becomes so severe that it is impossible to keep down any food or drink all day. That rarely happens, but when it does, the woman should contact her doctor or nurse.

Heartburn and indigestion

Later in pregnancy a woman may notice some other changes in the way her intestinal system functions. Women who have never had any digestive problems may find themselves having indigestion. This is because a muscle located at the beginning of the stomach relaxes. Normally this muscle keeps the contents of the stomach from returning to the esophagus. When it relaxes, partly digested food in the stomach can back up into the esophagus where it causes a burning sensation, often referred to as *heartburn*. Some steps which help to prevent it are avoiding fried, fatty or very spicy foods and eating light meals with snacks between meals. Some women find that certain other foods bother them. In that case, it's only common sense not to eat those foods. Avoiding lying down right after meals is also helpful; when you are upright, gravity helps to keep the food in the stomach where it belongs. If these simple measures are not enough, antacid medication can be used. Before taking antacids, or any medication, it is wise for a woman to discuss the choice of product and the dose with her medical adviser.

Constipation

As pregnancy progresses, the growing uterus presses on the intestine. This dislocation can lead to constipation. Drinking a glass of prune juice is an old-fashioned remedy that still works. It helps, too, to eat plenty of fiber from whole grains, legumes, and fruits and vegetables and drink lots of fluid. If these simple measures don't suffice, the next step is a conversation with the doctor or nurse.

Food cravings and aversions

Food preferences may change during pregnancy. Indeed, there is a whole folklore about pregnant women craving strange foods or combinations of foods. The reason for these unusual desires is a mystery. They certainly don't predict anything about the health or sex of the baby, as some old wives' tales suggest. And if eating a particular food will make a pregnant woman happy, why not? There is no harm at all in indulging food cravings as long as they don't interfere with eating well.

Sometimes, women find themselves craving things that are not food, such as laundry starch, clay, or ice. No one knows just why this happens, although one theory says that it is more likely to occur in women whose iron levels are low. (It's another argument for taking prescribed iron supplements.) Eating ice is harmless, as is eating starch, except for the calories it adds. Clay, on the other hand, can interfere with the absorption of nutrients. If cravings for non-food items get out of hand, it's worth mentioning at your next check-up.

Pregnant women may also suddenly dislike foods that they usually enjoy. This, too, has no significance. The simplest solution is to eat those good foods that do appeal, knowing that tastes will return to normal after the baby is born.

Breastfeeding

One of the first big decisions a mother makes is how she will feed her baby. This, too, is a subject about which pregnant women often hear conflicting and confusing advice. And on this subject, too, fashions have changed. For most of human history, there was no real choice and all babies were breastfed. Then in the 20th century, bottle feeding with more "scientific" infant formulas became popular and breastfeeding went into decline in the industrialized countries. In more recent years, science—and mothers—have found advantages in breastfeeding, and it is now coming back into style. It should be noted here that bottle feeding can be perfectly satisfactory and that the woman who chooses to bottle-feed her baby need not feel guilty about it.

Breastfeeding, though, does have advantages for both the baby and the mother. Human milk is the food most precisely designed for the needs of infants. Its composition changes as the baby develops to keep pace with its growth and requirements. In addition to its nutrients, breast milk contains immune factors which give the baby greater resistance to disease.

For the mother, breastfeeding offers convenience. The milk is there and ready without preparation or heating, a particular advantage at two o'clock in the morning! The woman who nurses her baby may also find it easier to get back to her pre-pregnant weight, since she is using up the energy she stored as fat during pregnancy. Finally, but very important, women who breastfeed their babies *enjoy it*. Nursing gives them a built-in time to sit down with the baby, relax, and share a special intimacy together.

Women who work outside their homes can still consider breastfeeding. During the time they spend on maternity leave, there is no problem at all. Even after returning to work, many mothers nurse their babies in the mornings and evenings, relying on a bottle for daytime feeding while they are away. And a few are fortunate enough to have child care facilities so convenient that they can feed the baby during the day.

Women who do choose to breastfeed their babies need to adjust their own eating pattern to provide the extra nutrients that go into the milk. The average newborn baby needs about 600 calories per day. To make 600 calories' worth of milk, a woman needs about 750 extra calories in her diet. That amount of milk will contain approximately 10 grams of the very highest quality protein. To insure that there is no drain on her own store of protein, the nursing mother's RDA for protein is increased by 20 grams. The table on Page 78 shows the recommended adjustments in the RDAs for vitamins and minerals to provide optimal nutrition during breastfeeding.

In addition to energy, protein, vitamins and minerals, a woman who is breastfeeding needs a liberal fluid intake. Two to three quarts of milk, juices, water, and other beverages each day supply the water that is needed to make breast milk. It's a good idea to have one quart of that requirement as milk and milk beverages which are a good source of the protein, calcium and other nutrients that are so important at this time.

To put it in practical, menu terms, this means making just a few simple additions to the meal pattern suggested for pregnancy. An extra glass of milk and three or four cups of other beverages will take care of the essentials. Some women will need more calories than that, but for most women finding calorie sources is hardly a problem.

A question that is often asked is whether a nursing mother needs to eliminate anything from her diet. It is true that what a woman eats can cross into her milk, but there is nothing in an ordinary diet that must be excluded because of the baby. On the other hand, occasionally a mother will notice that the baby seems uncomfortable after nursing when she has eaten a particular food. If that happens, it makes sense for her to avoid that food.

Drugs, too, may find their way into breast milk, so a woman who is breastfeeding needs to be careful about medicines. It is a good idea to check with the doctor or nurse who is caring for the baby before taking any type of medication.

There is one more point to consider when starting to breastfeed. While breastfeeding is a most natural practice, there are techniques which first-time mothers need to learn. This is easier for some women than for others. If getting started at breastfeeding proves difficult, guidance from a nurse or experienced mother can be a big help. With the assistance she needs, virtually any woman can breastfeed successfully.

Recommended Nutrient Intakes for Adolescent, Adult, Pregnant and Breastfeeding Women*

Nutrient (units)	Adolescent	Adult	Pregnant	Breastfeeding
Protein (grams)	46	44	+30	20
Vitamin A (mcg retinol equivalent)	800	800	+200	+400
Vitamin D (mcg)	10	7.5–5	+5	+5
Vitamin E (mg α tocopherol equivalent)	8	8	+2	+3
Vitamin C (mg)	50–60	60	+20	+30
Thiamin (mg)	1.1	1.0–1.1	+0.4	+0.5
Riboflavin (mg)	1.3	1.2–1.3	+0.3	+0.5
Niacin (mg)	14–15	13–14	+2	+5
Vitamin B6 (mg)	1.8–2.0	2.0	+0.6	+0.5
Folacin (mcg)	400	400	+400	+100
Vitamin B12 (mcg)	3.0	3.0	+1.0	+1.0
Calcium (mg)	1200	800	+400	+400
Phosphorus (mg)	1200	800	+400	+400
Magnesium (mg)	300	300	+150	+150
Iron (mg)	18	18	**	**
Zinc (mg)	15	15	+5	+10
Iodine (mcg)	150	150	+25	+50

* Food and Nutrition Board, National Research Council: Recommended Dietary Allowances, 9th revised edition, Washington, D.C., National Academy of Sciences, 1980.

** The increased requirements in pregnancy cannot be met by diet and require supplementation. Continued supplements are advised during breastfeeding.

10
THE AGING WOMAN

The fact that the American population is growing older is no longer news. This increase in the number of older people has created a new interest in their needs—as well as a vocabulary of euphemisms to identify them. Since aging is a normal, inevitable and honorable process that we all experience, this chapter will make no attempt to "prettify" the language in its discussion of the nutritional needs of women as they go through and beyond the menopause.

One growing area of research in aging is the nutritional needs of older people. Our present knowledge of nutrient requirements is based on research conducted mainly in young adults. From this information, nutritionists estimate the requirements of older adults. As we learn more about the biological changes that take place with aging, we will also understand changing nutritional needs. In the meantime, we can make some general recommendations based on what is now known.

Energy

The need for energy falls gradually after early adulthood. Several factors contribute to this decrease. The basal metabolic rate, the measure of the energy required to sustain basic life processes, declines with age; and most people diminish their physical activity as the years go by. In addition, older bodies have somewhat less lean tissue than the young, and it is lean tissue that uses the most energy.

The net result of these changes is a drop in energy requirement which reaches about 10 per cent after the age of 50, and 20 to 25 per cent in the 70s. Obviously, these are average values. At any age, an average reflects an approximate figure for members of a group and does not necessarily apply to any one individual in the group. Realizing this is especially important when dealing with an older population, because the differences between individuals tend to increase with time and age. Any woman's energy need will be affected by her state of health and vigor and her daily habits, particularly her levels of activity and exercise.

Minerals

Women who are menstruating need extra *iron* to replace that which is lost each month in the menstrual flow. When menstruation ceases, a woman needs only enough iron to cover ordinary wear and tear of the body. In terms of the RDA, that means a drop from 18 to 10 milligrams per day.

The RDA for *calcium* is unchanged throughout adulthood, however many experts believe that it is too low and that a more generous intake of calcium will help to prevent osteoporosis. Rather than the 800 milligrams of the RDA, they suggest 1000 to 1200 milligrams before menopause, and up to 1500 milligrams afterwards.

Sources of calcium are listed in Chapter 5 on Minerals, and in Chapter 8, The Adult Woman. To put it briefly, most American women consume 400 to 500 milligrams of calcium each day. To reach the 1000 to 1500 milligrams which are recommended to protect against bone loss, women need to use more high calcium foods, primarily milk and dairy products. Even with a good diet, calcium intake may be lower than is desirable, and supplements of 500 to 1200 milligrams of calcium may be needed to reach the recommended level. (See Chapter 8 for a discussion of calcium supplementation.)

Other nutrients

Recommended intakes of protein, vitamins and minerals other than iron and calcium remain unchanged throughout adulthood.

The older woman, as far as is known today, needs about the same amounts of nutrients as she did during her middle years. At the same time, though, her need for energy has decreased. It follows, then, that older women should choose their food carefully to obtain all of their nutrients without running their calorie intake too high. In practice that means choosing good food, fruits and vegetables, whole grain cereals and baked goods, milk and dairy products, and meat, fish, poultry, eggs and legumes, and going easy on high calorie items such as pastries, candy and fried foods. This sort of diet is good for women - and men - of any age; the only difference for the older person is the need for slightly more attention to limiting foods that provide more energy than other nutrients.

Symptoms of menopause

Many nutrition books mention the menopause only in relation to its effect on iron requirements; they ignore the hot flashes and other symptoms which often accompany the end of menstruation. The reason for this is that the symptoms of menopause are related to decreasing levels of estrogen, one of the female sex hormones, and not to nutrition. Nonetheless, some women find that their hot flashes diminish when they eliminate caffeine, sugar and alcohol from their diets. There is, at present, no good scientific explanation for this effect, but abstaining from caffeine, sugar and alcohol is safe and easy to try.

You may see or hear reports of one or another vitamin, most often vitamin E or one of the B complex, doing wonderful things for menopausal women. Unfortunately, these reports are based on anecdotes and individual experiences rather than on good research. It is an area that needs more investigation, but at present, there is no scientific evidence to support the use of vitamins to treat menopausal symptoms.

Osteoporosis

One problem of older women which clearly is related to nutrition is osteoporosis, the loss of bone with age. (Men also suffer from osteoporosis but at a much lower rate than women.) After middle age, the body loses the ability to maintain its fine balance between building up and breaking down bone. The formation of bone doesn't quite keep up with its destruction, so there is a net loss. The analogy of a bank account was used in Chapter 5 to explain the dynamic state of the skeleton, with minerals constantly being deposited in and withdrawn from the bones. To use the same analogy in describing osteoporosis, the withdrawals become greater than the deposits and the balance gradually gets lower and lower. As the amount of bone decreases, the skeleton becomes fragile and breaks more easily. That is why women with osteoporosis are so susceptible to fractures and why so many older women suffer broken hips and fractured vertebrae.

Some degree of bone loss takes place in all adults, beginning around the age of 35 or 40. In women, the process accelerates with the menopause, when lower estrogen levels lead to less efficient use of calcium. Osteoporosis may or may not become severe enough to cause a woman to have problems with broken bones. The progress of the disease depends on a number of genetic, nutritional, hormonal and mechanical factors.

Each woman's genetic make-up can affect both how her body uses calcium and how much bone she is able to make. Bones begin to form before birth and continue to grow in size and mineral content through adolescence. The skeleton is at the peak of its development in early adulthood. As bone is gradually lost in later years, the amount of bone tissue remaining depends on how much was there at the maximum, as well as on the rate of loss. Thus a woman who had a large amount of bone when she was in her 20s can lose more in her 50s and 60s without her bones becoming dangerously weak than can a woman who had less bone when she was young.

Nutrition is important at all ages in preventing osteoporosis. The maximum size that a child's bones can attain is determined by genetic factors, but whether she will reach that maximum depends on the environment. Nutrition, especially calcium and vitamin D, plays an important role in enabling the skeleton to reach its full potential. After the growth of the skeleton is complete, a generous intake of calcium helps a young woman to maintain it. And in later years, consuming large amounts of calcium (1500 milligrams per day) slows the rate of bone loss.

The absorption of calcium and its use in the body are regulated by an elaborate system of hormonal controls. Estrogen is part of the system. One effect of the decline in estrogen level at menopause is decreased absorption of calcium from the intestine. This, and other effects lowered estrogen may have on calcium metabolism, contributes to the development of osteoporosis.

Two strategies have been employed to combat the effects of diminished estrogen levels. One, which has been used to treat other symptoms of the menopause as well, is *estrogen replacement*. The therapeutic use of estrogen preparations will stop the progression of osteoporosis and may even produce slight improvement in the health of the bones. Unfortunately, estrogen replacement also appears to increase the risk of cancer of the endometrium, the lining of the uterus, and cause such annoying side effects as fluid retention and breast enlargement. By using a second hormone, a progestin, with the estrogen, the risk of cancer can be reduced. The risks of estrogen use and its benefits are something a woman should discuss with her physician if hormone treatment is being considered.

The other strategy which can be used to compensate for the less efficient utilization of calcium is to *increase calcium intake*. Even though calcium absorption has slowed down, if more is available, then more will be absorbed and used by the body. Vitamin D is needed to use calcium properly, but a good diet and some exposure to sunlight will provide all that most adults require. And since an excess of vitamin D is toxic, a supplement should only be taken under medical supervision. (See Chapter 8 for a discussion of calcium sources and supplements.)

Fluoride seems to strengthen bones and may some day prove helpful in treating osteoporosis. Research is currently under way but the results are not yet in.

Dietary protein, caffeine and alcohol can also influence calcium balance. High levels of any of those substances will cause the body to excrete more calcium, leaving less to remain in the bones. That doens't mean that they need to be eliminated from the diet but that they should be taken in moderation. Protein, of course, is essential, but most Americans eat far more than they need. Two glasses of milk and six ounces of meat or meat alternates provide a full day's allowance of protein for an adult woman. Unlike protein, tea, coffee and alcohol serve no nutritional purpose but most women enjoy them. There is no need to give them up entirely but there are good reasons to limit the amounts imbibed. An easy way to decrease caffeine intake is to switch to decaffeinated coffee and tea.

Smoking cigarettes, too, contributes to osteoporosis. No one knows just how tobacco works its effect on bones but it does. So this counts as one more argument against smoking.

In addition to genetic factors, exercise influences the amount of bone tissue. The scientific term is *mechanical loading*; what it means is that the stress placed on a bone when it is used in physical activity helps to stimulate bone formation. When the skeleton is not involved in doing work, as when someone is confined to bed, bone destruction goes on at a more rapid rate than formation, and calcium is lost. Physical activity, on the other hand, encourages the development and maintenance of healthy bones.

Once osteoporosis has developed, treatment, whether with hormones or nutrients, can halt the process but not reverse it to any great extent. That is, bone loss can be slowed down or stopped, but the bone which has been lost is not replaced. It makes good sense, then, to try to prevent or minimize the loss of bone. Measures that will do this follow logically from what is known about the causes of osteoporosis. To summarize them: maintain a calcium intake of 1000 to 1500 milligrams per day by eating a good diet with generous amounts of dairy products and other high-calcium foods and, if necessary, taking calcium supplements; be moderate in the use of beverages containing caffeine and alcohol; avoid excessive amounts of protein; don't smoke; and do engage in physical activity.

PART 3
Nutrition of Women with Special Interests

11
THE ATHLETIC WOMAN

Physical activity is the "other" part of staying fit. Whether the topic at hand is weight control, calcium balance and osteoporosis, cardiovascular health or general well-being, exercise complements good nutrition in promoting health. More and more women are showing their awareness of the value of exercise by engaging in activities to build and maintain fitness. They are running, swimming, cycling, playing tennis, working out and doing aerobic dancing, to name a few of the most popular activities. Some are doing it just for fun and fitness while others compete in races, runs and tournaments. All of these active women know that the exercise is good for them, but they may not be sure about how it affects their nutritional needs or how to eat when they are competing. In this chapter we will consider the relationships between nutrition and athletics, particularly as they apply to women who engage in strenuous activity and competitive sports.

Exercise and nutrient needs

The most obvious effect of exercise on nutritional needs is the increase it causes in energy expenditure. The size of the increase varies, depending on the intensity of the activity and the amount of time spent at it. An "easy" sport such as golf has little effect on energy balance, especially if the golfer rides in a cart, whereas training for a marathon can double a runner's caloric requirements. Differences like this in the demands of exercise, as well as individual differences in the way women's bodies respond to the demands, make it impossible to recommend specific calorie levels for athletes. A woman's best guide is her weight. If she is maintaining her desirable weight, then her calorie level is right; if her weight is falling too low, then she needs to increase her intake to keep pace with her activity.

Protein requirements are not changed significantly by exercise. The steak and eggs that have been traditional on training tables are just that, a tradition, and not a response to any bodily need. If a woman is engaged in a body building or intense training, her growing muscles may need an extra bit of protein but the difference is so small that that she has no need to eat more protein foods. The RDA for protein permits a generous margin of safety and, as you recall from Chapter 3, most Americans consume well over the RDA.

A cluster of nutrients that have become popular with many athletes are the *B vitamins*. There is some basis for believing that very active people have a higher requirement for certain of the B vitamins, an increase which probably relates to the roles of thiamin, riboflavin and niacin in energy metabolism. Each of these vitamins is involved in the reactions that release and utilize the energy from carbohydrates, fats and proteins. As a woman increases her physical activity her caloric requirement increases and with it her B vitamin requirement. If, however, she satisfies her increased caloric need by eating more of the good basic foods—dairy products, enriched or whole grains, green vegetables and fish, poultry and lean meat—her B vitamin intake should keep up with the higher requirement. The extra high levels of B vitamins in high-potency supplements have never been shown to improve athletic performance.

There is no reason to believe that other vitamins, B12, C and the fat-solubles, are needed in larger amounts by athletes than by more sedentary women.

The metabolism of only one mineral, *iron*, seems to be affected by exercise. Intense training and endurance sports such as distance swimming and running often lead to a decrease in the concentration of hemoglobin in the blood, a condition called "sports anemia." Exactly how and why this happens isn't clear. It may involve an increase in blood volume, that is, a larger total amount of blood with the same number of red cells, and greater fragility of the red cells so that each cell survives for a shorter time. Whatever the cause, women, whose normal iron requirements are higher than men's, are particularly likely to develop sports anemia. Given the difficulty of achieving high iron levels in the diet on a regular basis, women who engage in these strenuous activities may need extra iron. A supplement that contains the RDA of 18 milligrams of iron should suffice. Larger doses are unnecessary and may be constipating.

Exercise does not change the way that *sodium* is handled in the body but it may increase sodium loss and therefore sodium requirement. The sodium lost in sweat becomes significant when the activity is vigorous enough to cause profuse sweating. Even heavy losses, however, can be replaced by eating salty foods, drinking broth or bouillon, or adding extra salt to foods at meals. Salt tablets are not required and may cause stomach upsets.

Water

Even more important than the loss of salt in sweat is the loss of water. As in caloric need, the amount of water which will be lost is difficult to predict, since it depends on both the environment and the intensity of the activity. More intense exertion and a hotter environment both increase the amount of water lost in sweat. Although it is hard to estimate it in advance, it is easy to determine how much water has been lost by weighing yourself before and after exercising. Each pound of weight lost is equivalent to two cups of water. It is wise to drink an extra cup or two of water before starting a run or other activity which will cause heavy sweating. Smaller amounts, about a half-cup, can be taken at 15 to 20-minute intervals during the event and more at the end so that all of the water which has been lost is replaced.

A number of beverages designed to provide carbohydrate and replace the electrolytes, sodium and potassium, as well as water are on the market. Althea Zanecosky, a sports nutritionist and distance runner, has developed a formula for a homemade electrolyte beverage which accomplishes the same objectives, tastes better and costs less. Her simple recipe is to mix one quart of reconstituted frozen orange juice with three quarts of water and ¾-teaspoon of salt.

Diet during training

The best diet for an athletic woman while she is training is quite similar to the best diet for any woman at any time: a variety of good whole foods including fruits and vegetables, whole grains and cereals, milk and dairy products and fish, poultry and lean meat. The major difference between the athlete's training diet and that of other women is its caloric level. The athletic woman will need to increase her calories, using her best weight as a guide to the size of the increase. Most of the increase should come from eating more of the basic foods. That way, the amounts of vitamins and minerals will be augmented along with the energy.

Foods which are high in carbohydrates——bread, rice, pasta, crackers, legumes, fruits and starchy vegetables——are valuable in training diets. During exercise, the glycogen which is stored in liver and muscle cells is converted to glucose to be used as fuel by the working muscles. Eating generous amounts of carbohydrate enables the body to replenish the glycogen stores as rapidly as possible, within a day or two. If the diet does not provide enough carbohydrate, the glycogen level drops and endurance is decreased.

During periods of intensive training, a woman's caloric needs may be too great to satisfy without eating more high-calorie foods. Candy, nuts, cheese, ice cream and other desserts, gravies and sauces all add energy value. These, of course, are the high fat foods that should normally be used in only moderate amounts, but larger quantities are useful during periods of intense physical activity. Just be sure to decrease those items first when your activity level diminishes.

Carbohydrate loading

In an effort to maximize their glycogen levels before major events, some athletes go on a very high carbohydrate regimen. Known as glycogen loading or carbohydrate loading, it is designed to lay down larger than normal stores of glycogen to fuel the muscles during an endurance event such as a marathon, long bicycle race, or cross country ski competition. In sports that require short bursts of effort or are of low intensity, such as diving, sprinting, baseball and golf, glycogen levels are less important.

The principle behind carbohydrate loading is a kind of rebound phenomenon. When a muscle which has been depleted of glycogen is rested and supplied with carbohydrate, it will make and store unusually large amounts of glycogen.

When runners first started using glycogen loading to try to improve their performances, they often began with a very low carbohydrate diet, intense training phase. Most have abandoned that practice because the low carbohydrate intake coupled with the demands of training left them feeling debilitated. In addition, the sudden increase in glycogen was accompanied by an increase in the water content of muscles which could cause stiffness and a heavy feeling. Carbohydrate loading, as practiced today, involves a combination of tapering off the intensity of training while increasing the carbohydrate level of the diet. This approach works well without entailing the risks associated with intense training on low carbohydrate intakes.

A fairly standard regimen for carbohydrate loading goes like this:

day	level of training	diet
up to 7	hard	basic
6 to 4	moderate	basic
3 to 1	rest	high carbohydrate
0	competition	

A scaled-down version allows full training and the basic diet until four days before the event. On days 3 and 2, training is moderate and a high carbohydrate diet is eaten. Day 1 is a rest day with a continued high carbohydrate diet, and day 0 is the day of the event.

Successful athletes use both of these plans. The choice rests with the individual who can experiment to see which is most effective and most comfortable for her.

Eating on the day of an event

Pre-event eating should be planned to provide energy from foods that will be digested before the competition begins. That means primarily carbohydrates, since fat and protein stay longer in the stomach. Meal-time should be three to four hours before the event to allow time for the stomach to empty. Liquids move through the stomach more rapidly than solids, so liquid meals can be taken up to two hours before the event. Like electrolyte beverages, a variety of liquid meal products is available for purchase, but Althea Zanecosky also has a recipe for an economical, good-tasting liquid meal. She blends ½ cup of nonfat dry milk with three cups of fresh milk, ½ cup of water, ¼ cup of sugar and one teaspoon of flavoring.

Concentrated sources of sugar should be avoided during the hour before the event begins. Instead of providing a boost, sugar consumed too close to intense exercise can lead to low blood sugar and decreased endurance. That is because sugar stimulates the release of higher levels of insulin, the hormone that helps to remove glucose from the blood. Normally, when the blood sugar level decreases, the level of insulin also decreases and glucagon, another hormone, is secreted to keep the blood glucose from falling too low. Intense exertion while insulin levels are high removes glucose from the circulation too rapidly for the hormonal systems to adjust, and the blood glucose continues to drop to a level which will impair athletic ability.

Plain water can be drunk right up to the start of the event.

During and after the event

The only nutritional concern during the event is with water. If the event is long or the weather is hot it is important to drink some liquid, water or a dilute electrolyte beverage, to prevent dehydration.

After the event is the time to drink more liquids, of any kind, relax and enjoy your sense of accomplishment.

12
THE WEIGHT-CONSCIOUS WOMAN

We live in a truly remarkable culture. In many ways it is quite splendid but its influence on body weight and perceptions of overweight can pose problems. Consider the media. We are deluged simultaneously with messages telling us to munch, crunch, sip and swallow as well as messages telling us that "thin is in." Women's magazines seem to have recipes for rich, calorie-dense foods—and articles on weight loss in every issue. We are urged to splurge on enticing foods and inviting restaurants and then to buy high-fashion togs to wear while we exercise to shape up. And, of course, we need all sorts of labor-saving devices to free us from work and save time so that we can go to the gym or health club to work out! That may, or may not, be overstating the situation but it explains some of the concern and confusion about what desirable weight is, and how to maintain it. And it suggests why so many women fit the description "weight-conscious."

Desirable weight

The first decision which a weight-conscious woman needs to make is how much she wants to weigh. It would seem that it ought to be quite simple to find out or decide what one's "ideal" weight is. In fact, it may not be simple at all.

To begin with, there is a distinction between *weight* and *fat*. Overweight and overfat generally go together but the terms are not synonymous. *Overweight* means weighing more than some standard weight for the person's height. *Overfat* means having a percent of body fat which is higher than some standard. Most overweight people are that way because they are overfat, but this isn't always the case. An extremely muscular individual might weigh more than the tables indicate to be desirable and still be quite lean. There are several ways to find out how fat a body is. The simplest is to measure subcutaneous fat, the layer of fat just under the skin, with skinfold calipers, a device which looks something like the protractor you used back in geometry class. By grasping a double layer of skin and fat and measuring its thickness with the calipers, the amount of fat in the body can be estimated. This is done routinely in research on body fat, obesity and weight loss but has not caught on for everyday use. As a practical matter, most women judge by their appearance and, like most physicians and dietitians, rely on scales and recommendations for desirable weight.

That raises the question of why and how desirable weights are calculated. The purpose of height-weight tables and recommendations is to establish weight ranges in which individuals are healthiest and live the longest. The simplest rule of thumb is an old one that allows women 100 pounds for the first five feet of height plus five pounds for each additional inch. While this may be easy to remember and apply, there are no data to support its correctness. It is also obvious that women's bodies are too different from each other for any one weight to be best for all women of the same height.

The standards that are used most widely are developed by the insurance industry based on their knowledge of the heights, weights and longevity of life insurance policyholders. Some have questioned whether these standards are appropriate for the population as a whole, since individuals who buy life insurance may not be representative of the entire population. There is another complication in using the insurance company tables. Recognizing that differences exist among individuals of the same height, they list weights according to build, but they never explain how to determine frame size. In 1975, a government-sponsored conference on obesity simplified the table. This version gives an average and range of weights for each height and provides a reasonable guideline:

Desirable weights for height for women*

height in inches (without shoes)	weight (and range) in pounds (without clothing)
58	102 (92–119)
60	107 (96–125)
62	113 (102–131)
64	120 (108–138)
66	128 (114–146)
68	136 (122–154)
70	144 (130–163)
72	152 (138–173)

* from G.A. Bray: Obesity in Perspective, U.S. DHEW, Washington, D.C., 1975.

In 1983, the insurance industry issued a new set of recommendations which set weights somewhat higher than the old tables. The new standards have been criticized for ignoring health risks other than weight, specifically smoking, and for neglecting non-fatal health problems. The controversy illustrates the difficulties in defining ideal weight.

Despite these limitations, it is helpful to have some guidance in determining your preferred weight. It is well established that maintaining an appropriate weight is an essential part of promoting health. Obesity, which is correctly defined as an excess of body fat—but considered practically to be body weight of 20 percent or more above the desirable weight—is detrimental to health. Obesity increases the risk of developing high blood pressure, diabetes, heart and gallbladder disease, and some kinds of cancer, including breast cancer. A height-weight table offers an objective standard to guide women in avoiding obesity.

Estimates of desirable weight can serve another purpose. In addition to telling a woman how high is too high, they can tell her how low is low enough. We live in a time when the fashion is to be thin. (This hasn't always been the case—just think of the "full-figured" women in paintings by Rubens or Titian or even Renoir.) Models and movie stars set a standard of thinness that many women feel pressed to emulate; much of the anguish that women suffer about their weight comes from trying to conform to these media standards. We need to recognize the distinction between healthy weight and fashionable weight. Keeping to a healthy weight is an important part of staying well; reducing to a fashionable weight is an option which each woman should feel free to accept—or reject.

Energy balance

Energy balance, or the relation between the energy consumed as food and the energy expended in metabolic and physical activities, underlies the basic fact of weight control. If energy consumption is greater than energy expenditure, it produces a gain in weight; if energy consumption is less than energy expenditure, it results in a weight loss; if they are equal, weight remains unchanged.

In discussions of weight control, the term calorie is often used as though a calorie were some sort of material or substance (usually one to be avoided). Actually, a calorie is a unit used to measure energy just as inches measure distance and degrees measure temperature. The energy in foods comes from carbohydrates, fats, proteins and alcohol. Those food components can be measured in grams or ounces; the energy produced from them by the body is measured in calories. (Isn't it interesting that in food promotions, energy is often represented as "good" while calories are represented as "bad"?) In physics, a calorie is the amount of heat energy required to raise the temperature of one gram of water one degree centigrade. That is a very small amount of energy, so when we talk about nutrition and food we use calorie to describe what the physicist calls a *kilocalorie*, the energy needed to raise one kilogram of water one degree centigrade. (A small calorie is most properly spelled with a lower-case c and a kilocalorie with a capital letter, but in everyday usage, *calorie* refers to the large or kilocalorie.) Another unit for measuring energy is the *joule*. One calorie is equal to 4.18 joules. Physicists use joules to measure energy in various types of systems, and the unit is sometimes used to describe food energy or energy used by the body. (It's a term worth recognizing because it may come into wider usage, but we will stay with the more familiar *calorie.*)

Returning to energy balance, there is no getting away from the significance of energy consumption and energy expenditure, or calories in vs. calories out. We also know that there are differences in the calorie level at which individuals stay in balance even though these individuals may be of the same size and equally active. (But we don't know why this is the case.) We know, too, that for some people, regulation of their energy balance to maintain their weight is an automatic, unconscious process, while for others it requires continuous attention. Researchers are busily trying to explain these differences in the hope that understanding them will lead to better methods of weight control. Perhaps some day it will be possible to change a person's energy regulation, but in our present state of knowledge it comes down to decreasing the calories in and/or increasing the calories out.

Efforts at weight loss or control need to include attention to both sides of the equation. If calorie intake is excessive it should be cut down, but research on obese women has shown that they do not necessarily consume more calories than women of normal weight. Sometimes the difference between obese and normal-weight women is in their energy expenditure. If a woman is too sedentary, it becomes almost impossible for her to lower her caloric intake to the level that will maintain a good weight and here, increasing energy expenditure is essential.

Another fact of energy balance is the energy value of body fat, approximately 3500 calories per pound. That means that it takes a deficit of 3500 calories, or 500 calories per day for a week, to lose one pound of fat. With careful dieting and regular exercise, a woman can maintain a 1000 calories per day deficit and lose about two pounds of fat per week, but it doesn't take advanced mathematics to figure out that a woman is not likely to have a calorie deficit that will lead to losing much more than two or three pounds in a week. If that happens, as some quick weight loss schemes promise, what is being lost is not just fat—but water. This may happen if a woman cuts her intake abruptly; low carbohydrate diets are particularly effective in promoting the loss of water. The rapid drop that shows up on the scale may be impressive but it is only temporary. Permanent weight loss comes from burning up fat, not from getting rid of water.

Energy expenditure

The body uses energy for three types of functions: basal metabolism, processing food, and physical activity.

   1. Basal metabolic needs are the energy required to be alive, to support the ceaseless function of vital organs such

as the heart, lungs and brain as well as the biochemical reactions constantly taking place in every cell. The rate at which this energy is used, the basal metabolic rate (BMR), is controlled mainly by the thyroid gland. And we can't *will* it to change!

2. The second source of energy expenditure, sometimes called the specific dynamic action of food, is the energy required to digest and absorb the food that is eaten. Doing this work takes about ten percent of the food energy consumed.

3. The remaining way in which energy is expended is in physical activity. This is the one portion of the "calories out" side of the equation which is voluntary and which we can control.

Physical activity, of course, has benefits beyond its energy cost. The physically active woman has higher levels of HDL, the serum lipoprotein which is associated with a lower risk of atherosclerosis and heart disease. Her heart and lungs function more efficiently and she is less likely to develop osteoporosis as she ages. Furthermore, in addition to the energy expended during the activity, a 20 to 30-minute period of vigorous exercise raises the metabolic rate for the next twelve hours or so.

The choice of activity depends on a variety of factors, not the least of which is personal preference. For exercise to be beneficial, it has to be done regularly and a woman is more likely to be consistent about a form of exercise that she enjoys than one she dislikes. Some woman do well by joining an exercise group or class; they like the discipline of the schedule and the support of the other women. Others prefer to exercise alone, choosing the time and place they find most convenient. It's all a matter of taste.

How much energy is used in exercising depends on the type of exercise and the style of individual. Some average figures will give you an idea: compared to sitting quietly, playing tennis or walking briskly causes a five-fold increase in caloric expenditure, while running at a rate of 5½ miles per hour causes a 9-fold increase. Cycling at the same speed, whether outdoors or on a stationary bike, quadruples energy output.

In addition to sports and exercise regimens, there are ways to increase the physical activity involved in daily routines. The key word here is *walk*. Walk up and down stairs instead of riding elevators or escalators; walk, instead of driving, to do errands; park your car or get off the bus a short distance from your destination and walk the rest of the way there; at lunch time, take a brisk walk instead of sitting over a second cup of coffee. Any or all of these will increase your energy output without requiring any equipment, expense or special scheduling.

One note of caution: a women who is seriously overweight or who has any question about her health should have a medical check-up before beginning her fitness program.

Energy value of foods

Books and tables listing calorie values are easy enough to locate and use to find out how many calories are in a specific food. The intent here is provide more general information to enable you to understand and predict which foods yield more or less energy.

The first comparison to make is among the components of food which are used for energy: protein, fat, carbohydrate and alcohol. Pure protein and carbohydrate have the same caloric value at 4 calories per gram. Fat is more than twice as concentrated a source of energy at 9 calories per gram, with alcohol coming in between at 7 calories per gram. Water, which is the other major constituent of foods, provides no energy or zero calories per gram.

As you would expect from those figures, the higher the water content of a food, the lower will be its calorie value. Examples of high-water, low-calorie foods include salad ingredients like lettuce, cucumber and celery, other green vegetables and "wet" fruits such as melons and berries. As the per cent of water goes down, the per cent of carbohydrate goes up and with it the calorie value, so fruits with more sugar and vegetables with more starch are higher in calories. Then come the "drier" starches such as bread and cereals.

The proportion of fat in a food has even more effect on its energy value than the proportions of carbohydrate and water. Foods with even modest amounts of fat, such as poultry, very lean meat, eggs, and low-fat cheeses run higher than fruits and vegetables. Calories increase with increasing fat in meats, high-fat cheeses, pastries and fried foods and top out with pure fats like butter, mayonnaise and cooking oils.

Just paying attention to the way a food tastes and feels in your mouth can give you a good idea of its relative calorie value. For example, a small banana, weighing 100 grams (about 3½ ounces), yields 85 calories while a 100-gram, juicy, medium peach yields only 38. Again comparing 100-gram portions, celery (two large stalks) yields 12 calories; carrots (two small), 42 calories; peas (½-cup), 68 calories; and baked potato (one small), 95 calories. One hundred grams of white meat of chicken, very low in fat, provides 117 calories, dark meat, juicier because it has more fat, yields 176; and duck, the fattest of all, provides 310 calories. A 23-gram slice of bread comes in at 56 calories; a biscuit of the same size at 82; and 23 grams of chocolate cake at 100. Note, though, that 23 grams is an average size for a slice of bread or a biscuit but only about half of a normal serving of cake.

Beyond the calorie value of the food itself is the possibility of adding calories in preparing and serving the food. Any processing or preparation which adds sugar or fat to the food will raise its caloric value. To illustrate, a 100-gram portion of baked potato yields 95 calories. French fried, the same amount of potato provides 275 calories, and as potato chips, 578. The vegetables in a big green salad may be no more than 20 to 30 calories worth, but a tablespoon of salad dressing adds another 50 to 75. At a slightly different level, a half-cup of ice cream is 140 calories; two tablespoons of hot fudge sauce are 132.

Strategies for weight control

Any approach to weight control must recognize that, for those women who do not easily maintain their desired weight, weight control is a long-term proposition. It is not a matter of "dieting" for a few days or weeks but of developing a style of eating and exercising which becomes a way of life. The diet, a calorie conscious version of everyday healthy eating, has to be nutritionally sound and personally acceptable. One of the reasons why so many popular and fad weight-loss diets fail in the long run is that they are too far removed from normal eating habits; they may work for a while to take weight off but can't be sustained to keep it off. The "calories in" side of a weight loss regimen should provide adequate amounts of protein, vitamins and minerals, all of the nutrients except energy, while the "calories out" side should increase energy expenditure. After the weight loss has been accomplished, the calories in can be gradually increased while the physical activity is continued to maintain overall fitness.

Behavioral scientists have coined the term "self-monitoring" to describe the process of observing one's own behavior. When the behavior under observation is eating, self-monitoring takes the form of keeping a diet diary, a record of everything you eat and drink. If that seems artificial or unnecessary, stop for a moment and try to list everything you ate and drank yesterday. Even if you can recall all of the foods and beverages, have you any idea of the amounts you consumed? Recording each item as it is eaten is especially useful to identify the eating which is done almost without our being aware of it: the tasting while preparing food, eating the last little bit left in a serving bowl because it's too little to bother storing in the refrigerator but a shame to waste, and nibbling during some other activity such as reading or watching TV.

The format of the diet diary isn't important. What does matter is recording each item, including the quantity, when it is consumed. And don't forget the "extras," butter on bread or vegetables, dressing on salad, gravy on meat and the like. At the end of the day or, better still, the week, you will have a clearer idea of where your calories are coming from. If you want to be really precise, get a list of calorie values of food and look up everything in your record.

The diary now becomes a tool for changing your diet. First identify the high-energy foods which you really wouldn't miss—and eliminate them. Prime candidates for this would be snacks which you eat out of habit more than real desire. Next, look at the amount of each food or beverage. It's not uncommon for overweight people to choose their food well but eat such generous portions that the calories mount up. Half-cup servings of fruits and vegetables and 3 to 4-ounce servings of meat are considered by nutritionists to be standard portions. If you are eating larger amounts, try to limit the size of your servings, especially of high-energy foods. Finally, look for high-calorie foods which you can eliminate or replace with a lower calorie substitute, fruit or low-fat yogurt instead of a rich dessert, or graham crackers instead of pastry at coffee break time, for example.

Another use for the diet diary is to locate times or situations which lead to unnecessary eating. Realizing what is happening is half the battle. The other half is devising and following a plan for *change*. For instance, if you find that you nibble chips or cookies while watching TV, you might do several things. You could simply not have food in the same room as the television set or you could replace the high-calorie snacks with celery and cucumber sticks, or you could knit or do needlepoint to keep your hands busy while watching. Another thing which you might find is that you are using snacks as an opportunity to pause and relax for a few minutes during a busy day. In that case, you could just give yourself permission to take a timeout without having to eat or you could sip a low-calorie beverage instead of the high-calorie food. If your situation permits, you might find that a 10-minute walk does you more good than ten minutes of sitting.

Eating slowly is another strategy which helps to diminish calorie intake. Taking smaller bites, chewing thoroughly and pausing between bites all help you to feel satisfied with a smaller amount of food. That contributes to success in decreasing portion sizes. While cutting down on amounts of high-calorie foods, you can be liberal in your use of low-calorie items such as salads and broth-based soups. These take time to eat and add satisfaction without adding too many calories.

The technique of self-monitoring can also be applied to physical activity. If you find it difficult to increase your energy expenditure, try keeping a log of your activity. Include walking, gardening, climbing stairs and other routine activities as well as designated exercise. Keeping the record will make you more aware of how active or inactive you are, while analyzing it can help you find ways to increase your level of activity.

Cutting calories in food preparation

Having established the extent to which preparation can raise the caloric value of a potato, let's look at methods of food preparation which keep the energy value down. The most obvious is to refrain from adding fat. That means not frying, buttering or saucing with rich sauces. Alternatives to frying include broiling, baking, roasting, grilling, boiling and steaming. Pans with non-stick coatings can be used to brown foods without added fat. Potatoes, onions or other vegetables prepared this way won't taste the same as if they were fried with fat, but they will taste good and be far lower in calories.

Instead of putting butter or margarine on everything, be adventurous in using seasonings. Many vegetables are delicious when they are just steamed and served plain, but herbs and spices can be added to enhance or vary the flavors. People who are accustomed to buttered vegetables may need a bit of time but after a while they grow to appreciate the different taste.

Meat should be lean rather than heavily marbled with fat, and the visible fat on it trimmed away before cooking. Chicken and turkey are low in fat but can be made lower by removing the skin.

All of the fat should be skimmed off of soups and stews. The easiest way is to chill the food and then remove the fat which will have solidified on the top.

Low-calorie dairy products can be substituted for richer ones. Plain yogurt, for example, can replace sour cream on baked potatoes, in dips and cold sauces. It curdles too easily to be cooked but makes an excellent salad dressing when mixed with chopped scallions or basil, oregano or tarragon. Skim or low-fat milk can be used instead of cream in custards, puddings, quiches and sauces. Skim milk is less successful in soups but buttermilk has enough body to replace cream and adds a tangy flavor to the finished product.

Many recipes for baked goods and desserts call for more sugar than is really needed. In baking, sugar contributes to the texture and appearance of the product as well as the flavor but the amount can often be reduced by about one-fourth and still get good results.

Calories and supplements

Many women are concerned about meeting their nutritional needs while restricting their caloric intake. A balanced diet of 1000 to 1200 calories can provide enough of the essential nutrients and is realistic for long-term use. At calorie levels below 1000 there is more risk of inadequacy; below 800 calories a diet will probably lack sufficient vitamins and minerals. Very low calorie diets, 600 and under, are not only nutritionally unsound but risk causing severe problems and should not be used.

In the ideal world of nutritionists, even low-calorie diets are carefully planned and nutritionally adequate. In the real world of weight-conscious women, this is not always the case. Women whose calorie intake is below 1000 for more than a few days at a time are well advised to take a daily multivitamin-mineral supplement. Women who are less restrictive have less need of extra nutrients but may still prefer to take a supplement. In either case, a product which provides from 50 to 100 per cent of the RDA is suitable.

Smoking and weight

Smokers have been shown repeatedly to be thinner—but not healthier—than non-smokers. The risks to health of smoking are well publicized and need not be detailed here except to note that women are rapidly catching up to men in the incidence of lung cancer. *Not smoking is the single most important practice in health promotion.* The relevance of this to weight control is that a person who stops smoking often gains weight. Two factors contribute to this weight gain: a metabolic change which causes the ex-smoker to use less energy and a tendency to eat more as a substitute for smoking. Some women find their increasing weight so dismaying that they go back to smoking. From a health standpoint that's a poor trade. The five or ten pounds put on as a result of ceasing to smoke are trivial compared to the hazards of smoking!

A realistic approach is to be prepared for this to happen and take measures to counteract it. Increasing physical activity can compensate for the changed metabolism and keep a woman busy so that she misses the cigarettes less. In principle it is also possible for a woman to restrict her caloric intake to prevent gaining weight. In practice that may not work. For most people giving up cigarettes and restricting food alone are difficult tasks. Trying to do them at the same time may just be too much. It's reasonable to nibble on low-calorie rather than high-calorie foods when substituting a snack for a smoke but the best advice is probably to be patient and go easy on yourself. Take credit for the achievement of smoking cessation and wait until the craving for cigarettes declines to work hard on dieting.

Underweight

Most women who see their weight as a problem are trying to keep it down; some, however, find it difficult to stay up to a desirable level. Weighing less than the value in a height-weight table is not in itself a health problem but a chronically underweight woman should make sure there is no medical cause for her low weight. A sudden or unexplained weight loss is often an indicator of ill health and should be checked out by a physician.

Assuming that the underweight woman is in good health, what strategies can she use to increase her weight? It is not so simple as reversing the suggestions for weight loss. Physical activity has many benefits and should not be avoided; high fat foods need not be restricted to the extent that they are on a weight loss regimen, but should still be used in moderation, not excess.

There are some useful approaches, though. First of all, be sure to get enough rest. Although sleep has no nutritional value, fatigue can play havoc with a woman's appetite. For the same reason, be moderate about exercise; there is a difference between exercising to the level of fitness and to the point of exhaustion. Stress may have the same effect as fatigue. If stressful situations can't be avoided, learn to use relaxation and other stress management techniques to cope with it.

In choosing foods, select some that are high in calories. It's true that a very high fat intake is unwise, but jam and butter on your bread, cream soup instead of broth, and an ice cream cone as a snack are reasonable. There is no need to eliminate salads and low-calorie vegetables—you need the vitamins and minerals they provide—but don't fill up on them, either. Save space for the more substantial and calorie-dense starches and protein foods. Sweet desserts are a good source of energy.

It's easy to calculate a diet that increases calories by using large portions of food, but an underweight woman might find them unappealing. If your capacity at meals is limited, make a point of snacking at other times. Nutritious snacks include items like cheese and crackers, ice cream, dried fruit and nuts, cookies and milk, pizza, and sandwiches. Evening is a good time for heavy snacking because there is no concern about the snack decreasing your appetite at the next meal.

Sample menus

Here are three menus which illustrate ways to increase and decrease caloric value.

2000-calorie menu	1000-calorie menu	2800-calorie menu
Breakfast 　orange juice, 　　1/2 cup	same	same
cornflakes, 　　1/2 cup	same	same

2000-calorie menu	1000-calorie menu	2800-calorie menu
1% milk, 1/2 cup	skim milk	whole milk
whole wheat toast, 1 slice		same
		butter, 1 tsp
jam, 1 tbsp		same
coffee with 1% milk	coffee with skim milk	coffee with whole milk
Snack	coffee with skim milk	coffee with whole milk
coffee with 1% milk		
doughnut	graham crackers, 2	doughnut
Lunch	tuna salad platter	tuna salad sandwich
tuna salad sandwich		
lettuce and tomato salad	rye wafers, 2	lettuce, tomato and mayonnaise salad
1% milk	skim milk	milkshake
Snack		dried fruit and nut mix, 1 ounce
Dinner	chicken broth	cream of chicken soup
chicken noodle soup		
pot roast of beef, 3 1/2 oz	same, 3 oz	same, 3 1/2 oz
gravy, 2 tbsp	clear juices, skimmed, 2 tbsp	gravy, 2 tbsp
mashed potato, 3/4 cup	boiled potato, 1 medium	mashed potato, 3/4 cup
peas and onions, 1/2 cup	same	same, buttered, 1/2 cup
green salad	same	same
French dressing, 1 tbsp	herbed yogurt 2 tbsp	French dressing, 2 tbsp
roll, 1		roll, 1
red wine, 3 oz		same
Snack	same	banana, 1 large
apple, 1 medium		whole milk, 1/2 cup

13
THE VEGETARIAN WOMAN

Vegetarianism, the practice of basing one's diet on plant products and abstaining from animal products, is an eating style which has deep historical roots. Written accounts of meat-eating being forbidden date back to the Atharva-veda, a 3000-year-old Indian text. While the prohibition was based on the notion that eating meat was an offense against one's forebears, it also had the practical effect of protecting animals as a source of milk and eggs. Some 300 years later, the Jain religion was established by Mahavira, an Indian ascetic, partly as a reaction against the ritual sacrifice and caste systems of the existing Aryan custom. An important Jain belief is the doctrine of transmigration of souls, that humans may be reborn at higher or lower levels of existence. Thus even an insect may house a human soul and ought not be eaten. The same principle underlies the practice of vegetarianism in other Eastern religions.

At the same time eating meat was being prohibited as a religious matter in India, Plato, Pythagoras and their followers among Greek philosophers were advocating vegetarianism as a means of moral self-control. Avoiding meat was seen as a way of promoting the rational element in human nature.

Modern Western religious thought generally allows meat-eating and, in the Jewish and Islamic traditions, sets rules for the selection, slaughter, and preparation of flesh foods. In the biblical narrative, however, Adam and Eve appear to be vegetarians; it is only after the Flood that Noah and his family are given dominance over animals and permission to eat them.

Contemporary vegetarians

There are exceptions to the Western religious approval of eating meat. Most notable among mainstream denominations are the Seventh-Day Adventists, who include vegetarianism as part of their practice.

Other Americans, perhaps influenced by Eastern thought, refrain from eating meat because of a religious or philosophical aversion to killing animals as a source of food.

There are also vegetarians who have more secular motives for not consuming meat. In recent years some people have become vegetarians on the basis of their political or ecological perspective on food practices. They look at a world of finite resources in which many people are hungry and at the relative inefficiency of meat as a source of nutrients (it takes 21 pounds of protein in feed to produce one pound of protein in beef) and conclude that eating meat is a wasteful habit. Moving "down the food chain" in this view can lead to a more equitable sharing of the world's food supply.

Some vegetarians also believe that theirs is a healthier style of eating than that of meat eaters. Research comparing vegetarians with nonvegetarians suggests that this may or may not be the case and that each group of vegetarians or type of vegetarian diet must be evaluated individually. The one general rule that does hold is that the more restricted the diet, the more likely it is to be lacking in one or more nutrients. Thus ovo-lacto vegetarians, those who eat eggs and dairy products as well as plant products, are apt to have the least problem with nutritional adequacy. Next to them are lacto vegetarians, who consume milk and its products but eliminate eggs along with meat. Strict vegetarians, or vegans, partake of no animal products at all and need to exercise the greatest care to ensure that their diets provide sufficient protein, calories, vitamins and minerals.

Adequacy of vegetarian diets

The adequacy of a vegetarian diet, like any diet, depends on the specific foods that are eaten. Research has confirmed that vegetarian diets can meet nutritional needs for growth and development and for pregnancy as well as those of healthy adults. Studies of vegetarian adults have shown that they are leaner and have lower cholesterol levels than do meat eaters. On the other hand, there have been surveys of children which showed that the vegetarians were small in stature for their age.

The practical importance of these differing results is to emphasize that there is more to vegetarian eating than just eliminating meat. A vegetarian diet can be healthy and nutritious, but planning it——like planning any diet——requires knowledge, understanding and care.

Protein in vegetarian diets

Because meat is such an important source of protein in the diet, nonvegetarians are often unaware of the protein value of other foods. Eggs, milk and dairy products supply complete protein just as meat does. (You may want to go back to Chapter 3 to reread the explanation of essential amino acids and complete and incomplete proteins.) Among vegetable products, the best protein sources are legumes: soy beans and soy products such as tofu are highest, followed by other kinds of beans and peas, including peanuts. Grains, nuts and seeds also supply valuable protein. Other vegetables and fruits contain protein, but the amounts are small.

Even the best vegetable proteins are low in certain of the essential amino acids, which limits their usefulness if they are eaten alone. The limitation is easy to overcome by eating foods in combinations which, together, provide all of the essential amino acids. It's a matter of choosing foods with proteins which complete or complement each other, hence these combinations are called complementary proteins.

Grains, for example, are fairly good sources of protein but are low in the essential amino acids lysine and threonine. Milk is a good source of lysine and threonine, so the lacto vegetarian can simply drink a glass of milk or eat a piece of cheese to complement the protein in a slice of bread or other grain product. *Legumes* are also rich in the lysine and threonine needed to complement cereal protein. They are low in an amino acid called tryptophan and in several amino acids which contain sulfur, but these amino acids are abundant in grains. (The one exception is corn, which is low in tryptophan.) Thus combinations of grains and legumes provide more useful protein than either grains or legumes alone. It is interesting that in many cultures in different parts of the world, and going back far beyond our knowledge of amino acid requirements, food practices combined grains and legumes in traditional dishes. Examples of this include the rice and bean combinations of Latin America and the Caribbean islands, tortillas and beans in Mexico, soy and rice in the Orient, chick peas and bread in the Middle East and rice and lentils in India. Closer to home, the proteins in brown bread and Boston baked beans are complementary—as are those in bread and peanut butter.

Legumes and grains can be combined in many more ways: split pea soup and crackers; a salad including macaroni and kidney beans along with vegetables and seasonings, or a traditional Italian soup combining the same ingredients; soy flour mixed with wheat flour to make high-protein bread or muffins; or soy beans or chick peas puréed and seasoned to make a spread for bread or crackers.

Sunflower and sesame seeds are also rich in the tryptophan and sulfur-containing amino acids which legumes lack. They can be added to casseroles or sprinkled on soups to complement the protein in peas and beans. They also improve the protein value of corn and bean combinations. Tahina, the sesame seed paste which is a staple in Middle Eastern cooking, goes well in spreads and sauces.

It is clear from these illustrations that vegetarians have many options to consume adequate protein. It should also be clear that vegetarians, especially vegans, should do more than just eliminate animal foods. Some women, when they decide to change to vegetarian eating, simply stop eating meat and, perhaps, eggs and milk. They may just fill up on the bread and vegetables which used to accompany the meat. Women who do that risk an inadequate protein intake. A meatless diet can supply ample protein but it requires attention to alternate sources, dairy products, eggs or vegetable proteins selected for their complementary value. A good vegetarian cookbook might be a worthwhile purchase if you need more specific information about preparing these dishes.

Energy

Most of what we read, hear and worry about concerning energy is getting too much of it and how to cut down our calorie count.

Vegetarians may share the same concerns, but they may also have the opposite need, consuming enough calories. Not surprisingly, it all depends on their particular food choices. Fruits, vegetables, grains and legumes, the staples of vegetarian diets, are practically fat-free and therefore relatively low in calories. (A 6-ounce serving of steak provides about 500 calories compared to 200 in 6 ounces of cooked beans.) A lower calorie intake explains the tendency of adult vegetarians to be leaner than average but may also be part of the reason that some vegetarian children are small in stature.

On the other hand, vegetable oils fit into even the vegan food pattern, and most vegetarians eat dairy products which can be high in fat. More to the point, vegetarians are as varied as any other group in their use of fried foods, sweets and snacks.

In sum, vegetarian diets tend to be lower in calories than diets which include meat, but this is not always the case. Each woman can judge the suitability of her own caloric intake by whether she is maintaining her desirable weight. A vegetarian mother should also check with the doctor or nurse who cares for her children to be sure that the youngsters are growing at a healthy rate.

Vitamins

Vitamin D, riboflavin and vitamin B12 are the three vitamins which merit attention when planning vegetarian diets.

There is very little vitamin D found to be occurring naturally in foods. Small amounts exist in egg yolks and fish liver, but most of what we consume is added as part of fortification, particularly in milk and dairy products and margarine. Vitamin D is also made by the body when the skin is exposed to ultra-violet light from the sun. The vitamin D formed in the skin is usually sufficient for adults; only if you have very little exposure to the sun do you need a dietary source. That doesn't mean that you need to sunbathe, but just to be out in the sun as part of normal activities. Children, pregnant women and nursing mothers need more vitamin D and should have some in their diets. For lacto vegetarians this is easily provided by milk. Vegans can get vitamin D from fortified soy milk or supplements. A reminder: excessive amounts of vitamin D are toxic, so supplements should contain no more than the RDA of 400 I.U. (International Units).

Dairy products are the best sources of riboflavin, so this vitamin, too, is well supplied by lacto vegetarian diets. Green leafy vegetables; whole grain, enriched or fortified cereal products; and nuts are non-animal foods which contain riboflavin and should be used liberally in a strict vegetarian diet.

Vitamin B12 is the one nutrient which is found only in animal products. Vitamins are in plants because the plants make them for their own metabolic processes. Since they have no need for B12, they don't make any. It is made only by microorganisms in the soil and in the intestines of animals other than humans. Like vitamin D and riboflavin, vitamin B12 is supplied by milk and presents no problem to vegetarians who use dairy products. Vegans must rely on fortified products or supplements for their vitamin B12. B12 supplements, by the way, are made from bacterial cultures, not animal products, a distinction which is important to strict vegetarians.

Despite being water-soluble, vitamin B12 is stored and recycled in the body. That means that even a strict vegetarian who is consuming none of the vitamin may be able to go for months or even years without having symptoms of a B12 deficiency. This long delay might induce a false sense of security about the need for vitamin B12. But the effects of B12 deficiency are so serious—anemia and damage to the nervous system—that it is important to have an adequate intake and not wait for a problem to develop.

Minerals

This is beginning to read like an old refrain, but in mineral nutrition, too, vegans need to be considerably more resourceful than lacto vegetarians. You can probably tell from that statement that the mineral under consideration is *calcium*, another nutrient that is abundant in dairy products. Vegetable sources of calcium include sesame seeds, almonds, tofu, and some green vegetables: Chinese cabbage, kale, broccoli and okra. Other greens including spinach, chard, sorel and beet greens contain calcium, but they also contain oxalate, a compound that binds the calcium so that it cannot be absorbed and used by the body.

Most vegetarians probably need less calcium than meat eaters. As explained in the discussion of osteoporosis (in Chapter 10), people who have very high protein intakes excrete more calcium in their urine than do people whose protein level is more moderate. By avoiding meat with its large amounts of protein, vegetarians are less likely to lose calcium in this way and therefore may not need as much in their diets. The current recommendation that women get even more calcium than the RDA of 800 milligrams is based on the assumption that they are eating typical American diets. Our knowledge in this area is too limited to make a specific recommendation about calcium level for vegetarian women. It seems reasonable to suggest that vegetarian women who consume three to four cups of milk or the equivalent each day are probably getting enough calcium, and that those who eliminate dairy products should consider calcium supplements just the same as other adult women.

Iron, too, requires attention in the vegetarian diet and, for a change, milk is not a source of this mineral. In the typical American diet, meat is the major source of iron; its iron is absorbed more efficiently than the iron in other foods. Because vitamin C facilitates the absorption of iron from non-meat sources, the vegetarian woman can improve her iron nutrition by including a food which is rich in vitamin C—citrus fruits, tomatoes, berries, etc.—in the meal. Vegetable sources of iron include dark green vegetables, legumes, enriched and whole grain products and egg yolks. Soups and other foods which are simmered in iron pots pick up some iron during the cooking, so this is another way to increase the iron value of a vegetarian diet.

Zinc, like iron, is best absorbed from animal products and may be low in vegetarian diets. Most fruits and vegetables contain only small amounts of zinc, but vegetarians can get their zinc from milk and cheese, soy protein products such as tofu and miso, legumes and wheat germ.

One more consideration in ensuring that vegetarian diets supply enough minerals is the role of *fiber*. Large amounts of fiber can bind calcium, iron, zinc and other minerals and interfere with their absorption. In addition, phytate, a compound found in bran and whole grains, can impair mineral absorption. Phytate is broken down by yeast so it is not a factor in yeast breads, only in whole grain products that are not leavened with yeast or when bran is added to foods. This does not mean that vegetarians should avoid whole grains, only that they, like anyone, should get their fiber from a variety of whole foods rather than merely add extra bran to their diets.

14
THE WOMAN IN THE FOOD MARKET

The first step toward good nutrition is obtaining good food; it all starts on the farm and in the garden. Growing one's own food offers rewards of satisfaction, wonderfully fresh produce, and exercise for those who have the time, space, and inclination. For most women today, though, the starting place is in a store, whether supermarket, farmers' market or corner grocery. Let's look now at the concerns of the shopper as she plans and chooses her food purchases.

Information on the package

One good source of information about a food product is the package itself. The label must provide the name of the product, the quantity or net weight of the contents, and the name and location of the manufacturer, packer or distributer of the product.

Most, but not all, packages also list the ingredients in the product. The list must be in descending order: the ingredient used in the largest amount is listed first, the second largest is listed second, and so on to the ingredient used in the smallest amount which is listed last. A cereal, for example, which lists whole wheat as the first ingredient contains more wheat than any other ingredient. One which lists sugar first and wheat second would thus have more sugar than wheat in it. Coloring and flavoring agents may be listed simply as colors and flavors without naming the substance used. Should you want more specific information, you would have to write to the manufacturer and request it.

Some common products are not required to have a list of ingredients because they are covered by *standards of identity*. These standards are a set of government regulations defining the ingredients which must be included, may be included, and may not be included in a particular food. A product which does not conform to the standards must be called "imitation" or must be identified by some other name. Imitation mayonnaise, for example, is too low in fat to be called mayonnaise; low-sugar fruit spreads may not be labeled as jam or preserves. The original intent of the standards of identity was to prohibit adulteration of food products by spelling out the permissible ingredients. Contemporary consumers would probably prefer complete lists of ingredients, but the standards continue to apply to many products.

Nutrition information appears on many food packages. Federal regulations require nutrition labeling of all foods to which nutrients are added or for which nutritional claims are made. Nutrition information is optional on all other products. Whenever nutrition information is provided, it must be in a standard format. First the label must state the size of a serving and the number of servings in the container. It is important to take note of the serving size, particularly if you are using the information to compare different brands of a similar product. The regulations governing nutrition labeling say nothing about serving sizes, leaving it entirely up to the manufacturer. That means, for example, that if you want to compare the nutrients in two brands of frozen lasagne, you need to begin by checking to see what size portions the nutrition information describes.

Following the serving size, the label lists the number of calories and grams of protein, carbohydrate and fat per serving. The third part of the label gives the percentage of the U.S. Recommended Daily Allowances (U.S. RDA) for eight nutrients. The U.S. RDA are derived from the Recommended Daily Allowances (RDA), which are explained more fully in Chapter 15. The RDA provide desirable levels of intake for 29 nutrients. For each nutrient, the RDA are given according to up to 17 age-and-sex groupings. Clearly, the RDA are too elaborate and complex to be used on food packages. To keep the label readable, the FDA selected eight key nutrients. For each of these nutrients, they chose one value from the RDA, usually the highest value for adults, excluding pregnant and lactating women. These amounts of protein, vitamins and minerals comprise the U.S. RDA.

The information on nutrition labels is of limited value in meal planning, but many women find it useful in comparing food products. In making such comparisons, bear in mind both the lack of standardization of serving sizes and the fact that only eight nutrients are listed. If the eight nutrients are there as normal components of the food, the comparison should reflect other vitamins and minerals which are not on the list; however, this is not always the case. The label may be misleading if the nutrients have been added to the product. Then the food may be a good source of the added vitamins or minerals but not of the many unlisted nutrients which are still needed by the body. A simple example may make this clearer: orange-flavored beverages may contain even more vitamin C (listed) than is contained in fresh-squeezed orange juice but lack the potassium, folacin and other unlisted nutrients which fresh oranges also provide.

"Natural" and "processed" foods

We live in a world of growing complexity; technology increasingly pervades all aspects of our lives, creating problems as we enjoy its benefits. It's no wonder that in this milieu, anything natural has great appeal. Our food supply is no exception to this trend. The systems of food production and distribution rely on new technologies and leave many consumers wondering about the safety and nutritive value of their food. Some perspective is definitely called for.

Food processing refers to any procedure applied to a foodstuff after it is grown. Cleaning, trimming, peeling and cooking are all common forms of food processing. These and other processes, such as canning, freezing and drying, are needed to preserve and transport food and prepare it for eating. Their effects on the food's nutritional value depend on the processing and how it is carried out.

Drying, or dehydrating, is one of the oldest processes used to preserve food. Removing water from foods prevents spoilage and decreases the weight of the food, which can be an advantage in transporting it. (Just ask a backpacker about the relative merits of fresh and dried foods!) A newer method of dehydrating, freeze-drying, involves first freezing the food and then removing the water while it is in the frozen state. Freeze-dried foods retain their shape and, when reconstituted, have flavor and texture similar to the fresh product. Because the food is frozen and not heated, nutrient retention in freeze-dried foods is very high.

Like traditional drying, curing with smoke, salt and other chemicals is an old way to protect foods such as meat and fish from spoilage. In addition to preserving the food, salting and smoke-curing give it a distinctive flavor which many people enjoy. Recent research has indicated, however, that heavy use of cured meat and fish products may increase the risk of some kinds of cancer in humans, and that it is advisable to limit their consumption.

Using heat to preserve foods began in France when Napoleon offered a prize for the best method of preparing food for his armies' use. The winner was one Francois Appert whose invention, canning, has become the most common method of food preservation. The process is economical and does not require anything to be added to the food. However, modest amounts of vitamins are destroyed during the heat processing and more are dissolved into the liquid while the food sits in the can. The latter effect does not contribute to any loss of nutrients if the liquid is consumed.

Freezing offers the best nutrient retention of all of the current methods of food preservation, since the food is heated only briefly to blanch it, and liquid is generally not added in the preparation or packaging. Sugar is added to some fruits, however. Most plain frozen vegetables have nothing added to them, although a brine treatment used to sort peas and beans leaves a minimal residue of salt. Vegetables frozen in sauces tend to be high in salt and fat as well as price, all factors to consider in making purchase decisions.

Maintaining the quality of frozen foods requires that they be kept frozen solid. Thawing and refreezing damage the texture of the food and increase the risk of contamination. Food which is only partially thawed but still contains ice crystals may be refrozen. Food which has thawed completely should be either used promptly or discarded. It is good practice to thaw frozen food in the refrigerator or as part of the cooking process. Some foods, such as frozen poultry or shrimp, may also be thawed under cool running water but frozen food should not be left at room temperature to thaw. The surface of the food warms more rapidly than the inner portion and becomes a potential place for bacteria to grow and thus spoil the food.

Radiation is the newest method of food preservation and may gain economic importance in coming years. In this process, the food is subjected to radiation but, like a person receiving an X-ray procedure, does not itself become radioactive. The treatment has been proposed to destroy insects which contaminate grain, as well as to prevent sprouting in potatoes and onions. The safety of irradiated food is still under investigation by food scientists and by the Food and Drug Administration, which will have to give its approval before the process can be used commercially.

Food additives

Food additives are substances added to food products to accomplish some specific purpose. Many thousands of naturally occurring and man-made compounds are used as food additives; excluding salt and sugar, it is estimated that additives make up 7/10 of 1 per cent of the food we eat. These added substances serve a variety of purposes, including increasing nutritive value and preserving and enhancing the color, flavor, texture and appearance of the product. Additives used in food are regulated by the Food and Drug Administration, which is responsible for ensuring their safety. The Food, Drug and Cosmetic Act of 1958 established requirements for rigorous testing of all new food additives. It allowed, however, the continued use of additives which were used at that time and were generally recognized as safe. A list of these substances, referred to by its acronym as the GRAS list, was compiled at that time and the GRAS additives were not subjected to further testing. In the years since 1958, questions have arisen about some of the GRAS substances and several food colors have been removed from the list. Responding to these incidents and other questions, the FDA has asked the National Academy of Sciences to conduct a thorough review of the entire GRAS list and make recommendations concerning the safety of listed additives. That review is in progress and may lead to changes in the use of some additives.

Another possible change in the regulation of food additives concerns a provision of the 1958 law known as the Delaney Amendment. This Amendment prohibits the use in food of any substance which has been shown to cause cancer in humans or any species of animal. It was the application of the Delaney clause which led the FDA, in 1977, to propose a ban on saccharin, a ban which was prevented by an act of Congress. Critics of the

Delaney Amendment contend that progress in analytical chemistry in the years since 1958 now permits the detection of insignificant amounts of chemicals which would not have been identified when the law was enacted. Moreover, they say it allows no room for judgment or for the consideration of the benefits of using an additive or the risks of removing it from the food supply. Proponents of retaining the Amendment in its present form argue that it is necessary to protect consumers and that even the most minute amounts of substances which can cause cancer are not permissible in food.

The controversy over the use of sodium nitrate in cured meat and fish products typifies the complexity of the issues involved in regulating the use of food additives. Nitrate is readily converted to nitrite which, in turn, can combine with amines, compounds related to the amino acids in proteins, to form substances known as nitrosamines. Many nitrosamines have been tested and shown to cause cancer in laboratory animals; their possible role in human disease is unknown but the animal studies are grounds for concern. Based on this consideration alone, one might well wish to ban the use of nitrates in food. However, the reason that nitrate is used in cured products is that it inhibits growth of very dangerous bacteria, *Clostridium botulinum*. These bacteria produce a toxin capable of causing severe and sometimes fatal human disease; at present, no other additive is as effective as sodium nitrate in controlling it. Efforts are under way to develop a replacement, but it appears that eliminating sodium nitrate now to decrease a possible risk of cancer from food would increase the risk of botulin poisoning.

While the experts and the lawmakers explore and debate these issues, the consumer must choose which products to buy. While present regulation protects us from clearly dangerous substances, there are questions about the safety of some additives which remain unanswered. Each consumer will have to make her own decisions, for which the following suggestions may be helpful. Avoiding all additives and processed foods is neither necessary nor practical There are many additives which are truly noncontroversial, such as reasonable amounts of nutrients; herbs, spices and other flavorings; leavening agents; dough conditioners and some preservatives. Beyond this, be moderate in the use of processed foods containing artificial colorings and preservatives; emphasize whole, fresh and lightly processed food products. Eat a variety of foods to spread the risk. We usually think of variety as being important in obtaining all of the nutrients that are needed. In this case, variety serves to minimize any risk which might arise from ingesting a particular food or product by avoiding unduly large amounts of any one item.

Following the last recommendation confers an added benefit. Apart from additives, there are small amounts of potentially toxic materials naturally present in foods. Varying our food choices protects us from any risk which might arise from these substances, too.

Economy in food buying

As food prices increase so does a woman's interest in buying as economically as possible. The first key to economizing on food expenditures is planning - planning the budget, meals and purchasing. Planning a food budget means knowing how much you want to spend on food and keeping to that amount. If you are one of the many women who really don't know how much they spend on food, you might find it interesting to record all of your food expenditures for a period of several weeks. If the sum is higher than you would like it to be, analyze where the money is going and look for ways to cut down on the high-price categories.

Planning meals helps to ensure a balanced diet while using resources, including time, efficiently. It enables you to cook for several meals at one time and to make good use of leftovers. For example, you could roast a chicken which is large enough for two meals, serve it plain when it is freshly cooked and then make chicken salad, curry or a chicken and pasta dish another night. If you pack lunches for yourself or other family members, your plan might include leftovers to make into sandwich fillings or pack in insulated containers for later use.

Planning your shopping trip with a list saves both money and time. Although you might think your food will cost the same whether or not you have a list in hand when you enter the market, a shopper with a list is much less susceptible to impulse buying, picking up something which is not needed just because it's placed in a prime location. Time is saved because you can move through the store without having to stop and ponder as you go. You are also less likely to forget something and have to make another trip to the store to buy it, if you shop with a list. A convenient system is to keep a notepad in the kitchen and jot down items which you need as you are aware of them. That way the list is half finished when you begin to plan. It's wise to remember that the list is a guide, not an absolute rule, and to be flexible if an item on the list is unavailable, of poor quality, or priced very high. And the list should not keep you from taking advantage of other items which are particularly good buys, provided that you can use them. A sale item is no bargain if it sits on the shelf and never gets used.

Similarly, using manufacturers' and store coupons offers a saving if the product is one which you would normally buy and use.

Fruits and vegetables

In buying fresh fruits and vegetables, the first rule of economy is to purchase only as much as you will use while it is still good. Produce which is in season is more economical than out of season fruits or vegetables. Air transport has diminished the seasonal characteristics of our food supply, making it possible to have a variety of fresh produce all year. The cost of this luxury, however, raises the prices of foods flown from distant growing areas. Frozen or canned fruits and vegetables are often cheaper than the fresh and are worth checking out.

In selecting canned or frozen fruits and vegetables, house brands and generics often provide satisfactory quality at lower cost than highly advertised brands. Grading of these foods is based on appearance plus such characteristics as color, size and uniformity, not nutritional value. Grade A may be preferable for uses in which appearance matters, but there is no need to pay the premium if the food will be cut up or used in a dish where its visual qualities are unimportant.

In buying frozen vegetables, plain vegetables are always cheaper than the elaborately sauced products. An extra advantage to buying the plain vegetables is that you can control the amount of salt and fat that are added. Prepared frozen products tend to be high in both.

Grains and cereals

Grain products are generally reasonably priced but there are several things to know in choosing them. First is the comparative nutritive value of whole grain, enriched and unenriched grains. *Whole grain* is the most nutritious; but when it is milled and refined to make white flour, vitamins and trace minerals are lost. *Enrichment* adds thiamin, riboflavin, niacin and iron to the flour to return it to the same levels of these nutrients as were present in the whole grain. Enrichment does not add any other vitamins or trace minerals or fiber, so that enriched white bread is nutritious but not fully equal to whole grain bread and cereal. *Unenriched* white flour, or products made from it, have no added nutrients and are considerably less nutritious than either enriched or whole grains.

Cereal prices are extremely variable. Instant hot cereals are more expensive than are regular cereals. Small, especially individual serving size, boxes are more expensive than the large packages, and presweetened cereals cost more than plain. Like plain vegetables, plain cereals have the added advantage that you can control what you add to them. While most cereals are enriched or fortified with vitamins and minerals, the amounts of added nutrients vary. Some have modest amounts while others provide the full adult RDA for many nutrients. The latter are usually more expensive and are equivalent to taking a multivitamin tablet with your cereal.

Another grain, rice, can also be found as whole grain (brown rice) and enriched or unenriched products. The relative nutritional values are the same as for different types of flour and bread. Instant rice and flavored rice mixes cost more than plain, regular rice. Flavored pasta mixes, too, add a significant cost for the seasonings which, like those in frozen vegetables, tend to be high in salt.

Protein foods

Non-meat sources of protein, such as legumes and nuts, are the best buy in this group. Of the animal foods, poultry is less expensive than red meats. Cut-up parts may be more convenient to prepare than whole chickens, but their price is higher.

In buying meat, it is useful to compare cost per serving, not only per pound, since the amount of bone and other waste varies with different cuts of meat. Prime meat is more tender and has more fat than lower grades. Choice is less expensive than prime and its lower fat content is regarded by many as an asset. The less expensive cuts of meat are usually lean and quite flavorful.

They are less tender than the costlier steaks, chops and roasts, but are very good when properly prepared in pot roasts, stews and the like.

There was a time when fish was a dependably low-cost choice. Its increasing popularity as well as higher costs in the fishing industry have caused its price to rise and become extremely variable. Frozen fish is often cheaper than fresh and, with modern methods of freezing, it is of high quality. Canned tuna is another good buy. Its price often reflects appearance rather than taste or nutritional value. The lower-priced fish is fine for sandwiches and spreads. Use expensive chunk tuna in recipes in which having larger pieces makes a difference.

Dairy products

Milk, too, is cheaper in larger than in smaller-size containers, but the best dairy buy is non-fat dry milk. When reconstituted, it can be used instead of fresh milk in cooking and baking. By itself, reconstituted dry milk has a characteristic flavor that many people do not like as a beverage; however, when mixed with an equal quantity of fresh milk and chilled, the flavor is improved and the cost is still less than that of fresh milk. You can also add extra milk powder to a variety of dishes to increase their calcium and vitamin values.

Processed cheeses, such as American cheese, are cheaper than natural cheese and just as nutritious. The taste and texture are different because of the processing procedure and the addition of emulsifiers to the cheese. Cheese foods and spreads contain more water than natural or processed cheeses thus are somewhat lower in nutritional value.

Convenience foods

Convenience foods are defined as products which are fully or partially prepared and which require less time and preparation in the home. We often think that convenience foods are always more expensive than similar foods prepared at home. In fact, a government study of 41 products found that half of them were less expensive than equivalent home-prepared dishes when the cost of ingredients, fuel and preparation time (at the minimum wage) were all calculated. When only the costs of the food were compared, 58 per cent of the convenience foods were more expensive. Some convenience items save both time and money. Frozen orange juice, for example, is cheaper than juice squeezed at home from fresh oranges. Conversely, peanut butter and jelly combined in one jar cost more than when purchased separately.

There are a few generalizations which usually apply and which are well worth repeating:

1) canned fruits and vegetables are cheaper than frozen, which are often cheaper than fresh;
2) homemade baked goods and desserts are cheaper than convenience items;
3) instant coffee is cheaper than ground roast coffee;
4) dishes prepared at home are cheaper than frozen dinners;
5) frozen-prepared dinners and main dishes are high in fat and salt compared to good home recipes. This is changing to some extent with the introduction of a growing array of lower calorie dinners and other products.

What all of this says is that the prudent consumer has to make her own judgments about the cost and quality of individual items as well as decide how much time she has to devote to preparing her food.

15
THE WOMAN AT HOME

Planning and preparing meals is an everyday task, everyday in the senses of both familiar and "day-in, day-out." It is a task traditionally assigned to women. Today, as sex roles evolve, the traditions are gradually giving way, although women still bear the major responsibility for decisions and activities related to food. We do it all so routinely that we can easily forget how important it is and how many decisions are involved. The woman planning menus has to consider nutrition, cost, the availability of particular foods and products and the time that will be required to purchase and prepare them. If she is cooking for family members or others besides herself, their needs and preferences also have to be taken into account.

The importance of all this careful planning lies in the role of good nutrition for promoting health, and in the enjoyment of good food as one of life's pleasures. To these ends, this chapter offers guidance in meal planning, some practical kitchen counsel, and menu ideas for women and their families.

Nutritional adequacy

The primary purpose of food is to nourish, so the first criterion in meal planning should be to provide adequate nutrients. Various guidelines have been offered to women to aid them in planning nutritious meals. The simplest advice is the injunction to eat a wide variety of foods. While this is good counsel, it's too vague and gives no information about how great a variety or how much of different kinds of food are needed.

The Recommended Dietary Allowances, the RDA, are at the opposite extreme. Since this standard is applied so widely and in so many different ways, it is worth digressing to consider the background and intent of the RDA. Historically, the RDA go back to the time of the second World War when the government asked a committee of nutrition scientists to develop a "guide for planning and procuring food supplies for national defense." The members of the committee studied the nutrition research literature, made the best estimates they could and, in 1943, published the first edition of the RDA. Recognizing that nutrition is a young and growing science, the committee knew that its recommendations would not constitute an absolute standard but the beginning of a continuing process. That process of reevaluation of the recommendations in the light of new and increasing knowledge has produced revisions of the RDA at approximately 5-year intervals. The most recent edition, the ninth, was published in 1980.

As the recommendations were being progressively updated, the uses to which they were put expanded. Beyond their original objective, the RDA came to serve as a criterion for purposes as varied as planning school lunches, interpreting dietary surveys, and fortifying food products. While they do provide a useful standard for these and other public health purposes, the RDA are neither intended nor practical for individual or family meal planning. The intent of the RDA is to set levels of nutrients which will "be adequate to meet the known nutritional needs of practically all healthy persons." In order to account for the differences in needs based on age and sex, the RDA are broken into 17 age and sex classifications. Furthermore, knowing that individuals differ in their nutritional requirements and in the efficiency with which they utilize the nutrients in their food, the Committee on Dietary Allowances tends to estimate on the high side for most vitamins and minerals so that individuals whose needs are above average will be covered. Understanding this enables you to appreciate the difference between the *recommended dietary allowances* and any estimate of *minimal daily requirements*.

The usefulness of the RDA for meal planning is also limited by the fact that the recommendations are listed as amounts of specific nutrients, while meals are composed of foods. True, it is possible in principle to calculate the quantities of vitamins and minerals in meals but, realistically, who is going to bother? It is far more practical to use a guide based on foods than to try to compute amounts of nutrients. The **Four Food Groups** which are probably familiar to most readers, are just such a guide. They offer a workable definition of variety and list numbers of servings from each group which will provide a balanced supply of nutrients. The groups, recommended numbers of servings, and major nutrients in each, are the following:

Fruits and vegetables
  four servings (½ cup)
    one citrus fruit
    one dark green or deep yellow vegetable
    two others
  sources of vitamins A and C, folic acid, riboflavin, calcium, iron and fiber

Grains and cereals
  four servings
    1 slice of bread or ½ cup of cereal preferably whole grain; if not whole grain, enriched
  sources of thiamin, riboflavin, vitamin B6, iron and fiber (whole grains)

Protein foods
  two servings (3 ounces) of meat, fish, poultry, eggs or legumes
  sources of protein, iron, thiamin, niacin and vitamin B6

Milk and dairy products
  two servings (1 cup of milk or equivalent) for adults
  three to four servings (1 cup of milk or equivalent) for children and adolescents
  sources of calcium, protein, riboflavin, niacin, vitamins A and D and thiamin

This outline provides the foundation of a day's meals but not a complete menu. The idea is to start with the four food groups and then add other items according to your preferences. In fact, some lists of the food groups add a fifth, fats and sweets, not because they are necessary or even particularly nutritious, but to acknowledge that the four groups do not include all of the foods that people eat.

The simplicity that makes the four food groups so easy to apply has led to some criticism of them. Critics claim that the guide is restricted to basic foods and ignores the combinations and mixed dishes that comprise an important part of our diets. In a literal sense that is true, but the ingredients of a combination dish can easily be assigned to the food groups. Pizza, for example, doesn't fit into any of the categories—but if you think of it as a crust with tomatoes and cheese, you have servings of grain, a vegetable and a dairy product. A Chinese stir-fry dish might contain two servings of vegetables and one-half to one serving of a protein food. Tacos include all four of the food groups: meat or beans for protein, lettuce and tomato for vegetables, cheese as a dairy product, and the tortilla as a whole grain. It's not hard, looking at foods this way, to fit most of what we eat into the food group framework.

Avoiding excesses and promoting health

Guidelines such as the Recommended Dietary Allowances and the four food groups were devised to ensure that diets provide enough of the essential nutrients. Preventing deficiencies remains as important as ever, but more recently attention has turned to avoiding excesses of some components of the diet. This reflects the fact that classical deficiency diseases are now seen infrequently in the United States while chronic and degenerative diseases, including heart disease, stroke and cancer, are commonplace. Dietary advice designed to help prevent these disorders has come from government agencies and voluntary health groups such as the American Heart Association and the American Cancer Society. (Specific concerns and controversies about dietary fat in relation to heart disease and cancer and dietary sodium and hypertension are discussed in Chapters 2 and 5.)

There are also highly publicized disagreements among scientists about some of these recommendations, disagreements which can lead consumers to despair of ever knowing whom or what to believe. The basis for these disagreements lies in the complexity of the causes of the diseases. In the case of vitamin deficiency diseases, the role of nutrition is clear, direct and well understood. In such diseases as cancer and atherosclerosis, nutrition interacts with genetic and other environmental factors, making it more difficult to identify and define its importance.

To illustrate the problem, compare the possibilities open to researchers studying deficiency diseases with those of scientists investigating the causes of cancer. To learn about a deficiency disease it is a fairly simple matter to put volunteer subjects on a diet which is deficient in one vitamin and observe what happens. After the effects of the deficiency have been measured, the subjects are returned to a complete diet, supplemented if necessary with the vitamin being studied and their health is fully restored. So long as the subjects are properly informed and their health is monitored during the experiment, there are few, if any, ethical or practical problems in doing this type of research. The cancer researcher, on the other hand, would neither want nor be allowed to try to induce cancer in humans. She can do experiments in animals but studies of humans must look at people as they are. This type of research which relates disease incidence to dietary factors can show, for example, that there is an association between total fat intake and the occurrence of breast cancer, but it cannot prove a cause and effect relationship. The only possibility for manipulating people's diets is to ask volunteers to eat in a healthier way. Research of this kind can be done, but it requires large numbers of subjects and long periods of time to see any results. Even then, the interactions of many other factors may make it hard to be conclusive about the effects of nutrition in humans.

Because of this difficulty in proving the role of nutrition, scientists reading the same literature can arrive at different conclusions about dietary advice. Some want to wait for more hard evidence before recommending changes to the public. Others believe that there is enough evidence now to support recommendations to reduce the risk of disease. There is a consensus among experts on two points—maintaining a desirable weight and being moderate in the consumption of alcohol. Obesity and heavy drinking are generally recognized as unhealthy so there should be no confusion about them.

On other aspects of the diet, the weight of evidence and opinion favor change, although dissenting views can be found. These recommendations can be summarized as follows:

Fat: Reduce total fat and saturated fat. In the typical American diet 40 to 45 per cent of calories come from fat. To reduce the risk of heart disease and cancer, particularly of the breast and colon, decrease fat to 30 per cent. (Some experts advocate an even greater reduction, to 20 per cent.) Because of its effect on cholesterol levels, saturated animal fat should be kept low. The data on cancer indicate that it is the total fat intake, not the kind of fat, which is important.

Cholesterol: A limit of 300 milligrams per day has been adivsed to reduce the risk of atherosclerosis. (The table in Chapter 2 gives cholesterol values for foods.)

Sodium: Lowering sodium intake by restricting the use of salt and salty foods will reduce the risk of hypertension.

Sugar: Limiting the frequency of eating snacks which are high in sugar and other carbohydrates decreases dental caries.

Cured and smoked foods: Use these foods in moderation only. High intakes of smoked and salt- or nitrite-cured foods are associated with increased cancer of the stomach and esophagus.

In addition to listing foods to be decreased, the recommendations on diet and the risk of cancer include some foods to be used liberally. These include:

Fiber: A high fiber intake promotes healthy function of the intestine and may reduce the risk of cancer. This can be done by using whole grain products and generous amounts of fruits and vegetables. It is not necessary to add large amounts of bran which may interfere with the absorption of iron, calcium and other minerals.

Vitamin A sources: Dark green and deep yellow fruits and vegetables, sources of carotene which is converted to vitamin A, should be eaten frequently. Vitamin A supplements may not have the same effect and can be toxic.

Vitamin C sources: Liberal use of foods high in vitamin C may decrease the risk of cancer of the stomach and esophagus. It is not certain whether this effect is due to the vitamin C itself or some other component of the foods, so vitamin C supplements may not be as effective.

Cruciferous vegetables: Cancer of the gastrointestinal and respiratory systems may be reduced by frequent consumption of these vegetables: cabbage, broccoli, Brussels sprouts, cauliflower and kohlrabi.

Applying the recommendations

Understanding what the recommendations are and why some are controversial should enable consumers to decide how to apply them to their own food choices and meal planning. A few more considerations may help in making decisions.

An arresting feature of these recommendations is that, although they have been put forth by different groups with focuses on preventing different diseases, they all point to a similar diet. There are some variations, of course, but no conflicts between them. Items like using less sodium or more cruciferous vegetables appear in some recommendations and not in others, but there is nothing in one set of advice which contradicts another set. Whether your primary interest is in maintaining weight, preventing heart disease or cancer, or promoting good health in general, you can follow the same meal plan.

Since the recommendations are all compatible with each other, there is no need to choose between them. The only decision is whether or how much to change one's diet. One thing to bear in mind is how much risk you run, based on non-nutritional factors. For example, if your parents had high blood pressure, you are more likely to become hypertensive yourself and should be more concerned about your sodium intake than someone who has no family history of hypertension. Similarly, if your serum cholesterol level is high or you have a family history of cardiovascular disease, reducing saturated fat and cholesterol intakes might be your first priority.

What does this approach mean for the woman who is in good health and does not have any of the other known risks? It means that these changes are probably less urgent for her but *not* that she should ignore the recommendations. For one thing, while some individuals are at greater risk for these diseases, no one is immune to them. Secondly, moving from a typical high fat, high salt, highly processed diet to one based on more fresh, whole foods is a good, healthy move to make. Even the skeptics have never found any harm to result from eating less fat, salt and sugar and more whole grains, fruits and vegetables.

As a practical matter, changing one's eating habits is never easy. Experience has shown that small changes are not as difficult to make as large ones, and that gradual change is more acceptable than an abrupt transformation. If the food choices and meal patterns that follow differ greatly from what you are accustomed to, the most realistic approach may be to choose *one* initial change to make. It can be as simple as switching from whole milk and cream to low fat milk, choosing whole grain instead of white bread, or seasoning vegetables with herbs instead of salt Persevere with that modification until it becomes natural-it will, if you give it time-and then add a second change, perhaps replacing red meat with fish or chicken for dinner once or twice each week or serving dark green vegetables more often. When the second change feels routine, then move on to another.

Some changes may be easier to make than others. If that is the case, start with the easiest ones and build on your early success. Eating habits are a long-term proposition; it is neither necessary nor realistic to expect to make radical changes in them instantaneously.

Food choices

To see how these recommendations can be utilized in making food choices, let's start by looking at the four food groups.

Fruits and vegetables: Use foods in this group liberally. There are no restrictions but some fruits and vegetables deserve special emphasis: carotene-rich dark green and deep yellow or orange fruits and vegetables such as broccoli, spinach, peppers, apricots, cantaloupe, carrots and winter squash; vitamin C-rich citrus fruits, berries and melons; and vegetables in the cabbage family.

Grains and cereals: The recommended four servings from this group may be more than many women eat, since concern about caloric intake often leads to cutting out bread. Whole grains, however, are an excellent source of fiber and should be included. Enriched grain products are equivalent to whole grains in vitamins and iron but lack the fiber and other trace minerals found in unrefined grains.

Protein foods: Selection in this group should consider the fat level of the food. Fish and legumes are the protein foods with the least fat, with chicken, turkey and veal close behind; these should be the items used most often from the protein group. Red meats, beef, lamb and pork, are higher in fat. They don't need to be totally excluded but should be used less often than the lower fat choices. Lunch meats, sausages and the like suffer from being both high in fat and salt and from being cured products; their use should be infrequent.

Milk and dairy products: Skim and low fat milk have all of the protein, vitamins and minerals of whole milk but less fat and thus are preferable choices. Similarly, low fat yogurt is better than yogurt made from whole milk. Cheeses, too, have varying amounts of fat. It is better to eat those which are lower in fat most of the time and reserve the very rich ones for limited use. Frozen yogurt and soft ice cream are lower in fat and higher in calcium than regular ice cream. Save the latter for occasional treats.

The *fats and sweets* which comprise the fifth group are high-energy, low-nutrient foods, reason enough to go easy on them. As we have already seen, a high fat intake is associated with a higher risk of heart disease and cancer and should definitely be avoided. Since the risk of heart disease is also affected by the ratio of polyunsaturated to saturated fat, it is a good idea to use polyunsaturated oils rather than solid shortening when you do use fats in cooking.

Food storage

The way in which food is stored in the home is important in preserving its nutritional value and wholesomeness.

Several of the vitamins, especially C, can be destroyed by exposure to oxygen in the air. The rate of this destruction depends on the temperature; the lower the temperature, the slower the loss of the vitamin. Other vitamins, such as riboflavin, are damaged by exposure to light; this process, too, is retarded by cooling.

In addition to preserving vitamins, keeping perishable foods, including meat, fish, poultry and dairy products, chilled will prevent spoilage. Bacteria abound in the world and there is no way to keep foods free of them. By storing vulnerable food products in a refrigerator at a temperature below 45 degrees Fahrenheit, the bacteria can be kept from growing and spoiling the food. Cooked food which is to be kept should be chilled promptly by being put in the refrigerator, not left out on a counter to cool.

Bacteria can't grow without moisture, which is why dry foods such as cereal and dry beans do not require refrigeration. They do need to be kept in a dry place, however.

Nuts and whole grain flours contain oils which can react with oxygen in the air and turn rancid. They are not spoiled in the sense of being dangerous to eat, but the taste is no longer appetizing. To prevent this from happening, store them in a cool place or, for longer storage, in the refrigerator or freezer.

Even dry and canned products don't maintain their quality forever. They can be stored at room temperature, but be sure to arrange them in the cupboard in such a way that what was bought first is used first. If you are not attentive, it's easy to put the new cans or boxes on the front of the shelf, use them, replace them, use the replacements and so on, while older packages remain untouched in the back.

While it is not, strictly speaking, a matter of nutrition or wholesomeness, another important practice in kitchen storage is to keep food and non-food products in their original containers. If there is a need to transfer them, be sure that the new container is clearly marked and that household products such as detergents and cleaning solvents are never stored in food containers. This is good procedure for everyone and especially important in homes where children live.

Food preparation

The preparation of food can alter its nutritional value by the loss of vitamins and minerals or the addition of fat, salt or sugar to the product.

Vitamins that are destroyed by light or oxygen during storage are susceptible to the same effects during preparation. In addition, these and other vitamins, including thiamin and B6, can be damaged by heat. While some loss during cooking is inevitable, it can be minimized by cooking foods just until they are done and not overcooking them.

Another way that minerals and water-soluble vitamins are lost is by dissolving nutriments into water which is then discarded. Nutrients leaching out into the water is no problem if the liquid will be consumed, as in a soup or stew. It is possible to save the liquid left from cooking vegetables and use it later in a soup or sauce, a practice which is often recommended but which many women find impractical. Another way to decrease these losses is to use an absolute minimum of water or to steam rather than boil the vegetables. Leaving the food in large pieces also helps because the nutrients are dissolved from the surface of the food. A whole potato, for example, has less surface exposed to cooking water than the same potato cut into small pieces. And if the skin is left on, the potato will give up still less of its nutrients.

These techniques of using a small amount of water and cooking vegetables rapidly and briefly help to keep the colors bright and the appearance attractive as well as to preserve the nutritive value of the food. Beware of one trick sometimes used to keep green vegetables looking nice which actually increases the loss of vitamins. Baking soda added to cooking water makes it slightly alkaline and the green pigments in vegetables stay very bright in alkaline solutions. It is possible to have overcooked, soft vegetables that retain their good color. But vitamins, unlike the green color, are less stable in alkaline solutions, so adding baking soda to vegetables decreases their nutritional value.

The method of preparation, as well as the ingredients used, affects the fat and calorie value of the dish that is served. To keep the fat level down, avoid frying or sautéing foods in fats or oils. Instead, broil, bake, roast, simmer or steam the food. Or "fry" it in a pan with a non-stick coating These can be used for preparing anything from scrambled eggs to hashed brown potatoes without adding any fat. Products cooked in them are not exactly the same as those made in the traditional way, but they can be just as good to eat and healthier, too.

People who are accustomed to using a lot of salt will find lightly salted or unsalted foods lacking in taste at first. Over a period of weeks or a few months, the taste buds adjust and most foods are perfectly acceptable without salt. To ease the transition, and add to the interest of food in general, you can use a whole array of herbs and spices to season without salt. Fresh or powdered onion and garlic, wine and lemon juice enhance flavors without adding sodium.

The same flavorings can be used to make vegetables taste good without added butter, thus cutting down on another common source of fat. Margarine, by the way, is made from vegetable oils so has no cholesterol, but *margarine's fat and calorie values are the same as butter's.*

Low fat products can also be substituted for richer ones in many instances. One of the most versatile is plain yogurt which can replace mayonnaise or sour cream in salads, toppings, baked goods, dips and cold sauces. About the only place in which it cannot be used is hot sauces because yogurt's acidity makes it curdle too easily when heated. If you find yogurt too watery for these culinary purposes, you can prepare thickened yogurt quite easily. Simply line a sieve or colander with cheesecloth (a paper towel will do in a pinch), set it in a bowl, pour in the yogurt and let it drain until it is as thick as you like. A half-hour to an hour is usually enough time to thicken it. Let it stand overnight in the refrigerator and it will become thick enough to spread on bread or toast as a low fat alternative to cream cheese.

Whole milk usually has 3½ per cent fat. Low fat milk is 1 or 2 per cent fat and skim milk has none, making them good whole milk substitutes. Powdered skim milk is economical, too. Its taste is not quite the same as fresh milk but it is perfectly acceptable in cooking or in coffee. To increase its calcium value, reconstitute the milk using 1½ times the recommended amount of powder. The dry milk can also be added to soups, puddings and casseroles to add extra calcium to the product.

Buttermilk, which is low in fat, can substitute for cream in some recipes. It works well in chilled soups, providing both a nice texture and tangy flavor.

If you bake, try using part whole wheat or other whole grain flour in recipes for everything except delicate cakes. The difference may not even be detectable in intensely flavored products like brownies or gingerbread. In other baked goods such as biscuits, muffins, cookies and breads, whole grain flours impart a flavor and texture which are often more interesting and appealing than white flour at the same time they are adding fiber and trace minerals.

Fresh fruit is the basic ingredient in many nutritious desserts. It's good simply eaten plain, as is customary in many European countries, or it can be made into fancier dishes. Pears poached in red wine, for example, make an elegant dessert. Fresh berries or other seasonal fruit can be topped with low fat yogurt sweetened with just a touch of honey. Sorbets and fruit ices are both fashionable and fat-free. So are meringue shells, which can be filled with any lovely fruit, and angel food cake, which can be served with a fruit and yogurt topping. Apple crisp, made with rolled oats and whole wheat flour, tastes just as good as apple pie, but has less fat and more fiber. These suggestions aren't meant to imply that healthy eating means never having fried chicken, potato chips, white bread or ice cream. There is no food which has to be given up entirely; it's a matter of *how much* and *how often*. Fried foods, salty foods, rich desserts and the like ought not to be everyday staples, but there is no harm in having them occasionally. It's a matter of balance and the long term.

Meal planning

Menus for breakfasts, lunches and dinners illustrate the application of these nutritional guidelines to planning meals and adapting recipes. A few comments about them are in order here. You may notice similarities between some of the breakfast and lunch menus. If that surprises you, it is only because we tend to be such creatures of habit about what constitutes breakfast food. Why not have some variety in the morning the same as you do later in the day?

The total calories and percentage of calories from fat are calculated for each meal. Assuming that any milk used has 1 per cent fat, the calories from fat range from 11 to 36 per cent, with most falling between 20 and 30 per cent. This allows you to have some additional fat, either in the meals or in snacks, and still be within the recommended level of 30 per cent.

Beverages are left for individual choice rather than specified. A glass of low fat milk, always a good choice, adds 100 calories and just a little bit of fat. Coffee and tea have no nutritive value unless you add milk, cream or sugar. (Using extra-strength skim milk is a good way to make even the amount in a cup of coffee a source of calcium and vitamins.) If you drink more than a couple of cups each day, it would be a good idea to use decaffeinated products at least some of the time.

Suggestions for preparing some of the main dishes and information on how varying the ingredients changes the nutritive value of the product are given in the hope that they will give you ideas for other menus and recipes. The goal is to plan and prepare meals that taste good and keep you well.

Breakfast

The first menu is based on a breakfast milkshake made by putting one cup of milk and a ripe banana in a blender with a pinch of cinnamon or nutmeg and whirring the mixture until it is smooth and frothy. As given, the meal yields 335 calories, 19 per cent from fat. If skim milk were used instead of one per cent, the calories drop to 320 with 13 per cent from fat. Using whole milk would raise the calories to 390 with 29 per cent from fat. Adding a teaspoon of butter on the muffin with the whole milk would yield 425 calories, 35 per cent from fat. Having the butter but using the one per cent milk, the meal would come in at 370 calories, 26 per cent from fat.

> banana breakfast shake
> bran muffin
> **calories: 335 (19 per cent from fat)**

> orange juice, ½ cup
> bagel, toasted with cheddar cheese, 1 ounce
> coffee with milk
> **calories: 345 (31 per cent from fat)**

granola, ½ cup
yogurt, 1 cup
strawberries, ½ cup
    calories: 410 (22 per cent from fat)

grapefruit juice, ½ cup
cottage cheese, ½ cup
blueberry muffin
coffee with milk
    calories: 300 (20 per cent from fat)

Lunch

Broccoli quiche is a good dish to show how a recipe can be modified to change its fat content. Let's begin with a standard recipe calling for a pastry shell, two cups of chopped broccoli, ¾ cup of shredded Swiss cheese, ¼ cup of grated parmesan, one cup of cream, one cup of whole milk and four eggs. The quiche is an excellent source of calcium, vitamin A and riboflavin and a fair source of vitamin C. Another plus is that the broccoli is a cruciferous vegetable. One serving of the quiche, however, has 355 calories with 63 per cent of them from fat. By using all whole milk, the calories are reduced to 305 with 56 per cent from fat. One per cent milk brings it down to 285 calories and 53 per cent from fat and skim milk to 280 calories, 52 per cent from fat. Reducing the amount of cheese would also reduce the fat and calories, but it would reduce the nutrients and flavor, too. You would probably prefer to leave in all of the cheese and consider the quiche as one of your high fat treats, saving fat in other places. Another possibility is to skip the crust and serve the filling as a broccoli-cheese custard. It's no longer a quiche, but it is still a good luncheon dish and has only 170 calories, 43 per cent from fat.

    The menu as given, with the quiche made with 1 per cent milk, comes in at 475 calories, 36 per cent from fat. That's over the target of 30 per cent, but this is only one meal, not a steady diet. If you substituted the custard version of the dish for the quiche in the same menu, the calories come down to 360, 29 per cent from fat. Another way to reduce the percentage of calories from fat is to eat the quiche and add a glass of wine to bring the total calories to 560 with 31 per cent from fat (but that's sneaky).

>broccoli-cheese quiche
>sliced tomato
>whole wheat roll
>fresh fruit cup
>**calories: 475 (36 per cent from fat)**

>mixed fresh fruit, 1 cup
>yogurt, 1 cup
>honey, 1 tablespoon
>graham crackers, 2
>tea or decaf coffee
>**calories: 435 (11 per cent from fat)**

>curried chicken salad, made with yogurt dressing, ¼ cup, on whole wheat bread, 2 slices
>carrot sticks, 1 medium carrot
>celery, 3 stalks
>orange, 1 medium
>tea or decaf coffee
>**calories: 300 (16 per cent from fat)**

>cantaloupe, ½ melon
>cottage cheese, ¾ cup
>bread sticks, 4 medium
>oatmeal raisin cookie, 1
>iced tea
>**calories: 395 (23 per cent from fat)**

Dinner

The dinner menus include main dishes which require more preparation and offer more examples of low fat recipes.

The first menu features a meatless baked stuffed eggplant. Most stuffed eggplant recipes call for cooking the eggplant in oil and combining it with browned meat. For this dish, partially bake the eggplant, cut it in half, scoop out the pulp and chop it coarsely. Brown it in a non-stick pan along with chopped onion, green pepper and garlic. When the vegetables are browned combine them with one cup of cooked brown rice, two ounces of grated cheddar cheese, one-half cup of ricotta or cottage cheese, a big pinch of dried basil and pepper to taste. Put the filling into the eggplant shells and bake until the tops are browned.

Low fat chicken parmesan can be prepared by browning a boned and skinned chicken breast under the broiler or in a nonstick pan, putting it in a baking dish, topping it with tomato sauce, an ounce of part skim milk mozzarella cheese and a tablespoon of grated parmesan cheese and baking it until the chicken is done and the cheeses melted. The result has 275 calories, 25 per cent from fat, compared to a standard commercial product which has over 600 calories and 43 per cent fat.

The meatloaf, or any dish made with ground meat, can be made lower in fat, and cost, by replacing half of the beef or pork with ground turkey. The calculations for the meatloaf dinner were based on using half-beef and half-turkey.

The last menu, with a fish main dish, is the lowest of all in fat. To prepare it, lightly oil a square of baking parchment or aluminum foil. Put a 6-ounce fillet of haddock or other lean fish in the center, cover the fish with slices of tomato and add a tablespoon of chopped onion, carrot and celery, some dried thyme and pepper. Fold the paper or foil around the fish and bake the whole package in a hot (400°) oven for 20 minutes. This dish is so low in fat that you could even have ice cream for dessert and still keep the total calories for the meal at 525, with only 26 per cent from fat.

> baked stuffed eggplant
> steamed peas, ½ cup
> French bread, 1 slice
> baked pear, 1 medium
> **calories: 610 (30 per cent from fat)**

> chicken parmesan
> whole wheat spaghetti, ¾ cup
> mixed green salad with 1 tablespoon Italian dressing
> Italian bread, 1 slice
> fresh peach, 1 medium
> **calories: 660 (25 per cent from fat)**

meatloaf, 3 ½ ounces
baked potato, 1 medium with 2 tablespoons thick yogurt
steamed broccoli, 1 large stalk
apple crisp, 1 average serving
    calories: 560 (21 per cent from fat)

baked haddock
rice, ½ cup
zucchini, ½ cup
cabbage salad, ½ cup
rye roll, 1
baked custard, ½ cup
    calories: 500 (15 per cent from fat)

16
THE WOMAN AWAY FROM HOME

The number of women who work outside of their homes and travel as part of their work continues to increase. One consequence of these trends is that women eat more of their meals away from home. When "eating out" was an occasional treat, the nutritional aspects of the meals commanded little attention; but as it becomes a regular part of many women's style of living, they have become much more concerned about nutrition when eating away from home.

Eating at the job

Break-time in many workplaces means coffee and doughnuts or Danish pastry. These may be all that the local coffee cart or vending machines have to offer. The woman who wants more nutrition and less fat often has to supply her own snacks. A piece of fresh fruit or a few crackers and a chunk of cheese can fit between the papers in a briefcase or in a large handbag, to be nibbled on at work. Another possibility is to keep good, nonperishable provisions on hand. Instant low fat hot chocolate is an alternative to coffee and tea; graham crackers taste good and contain more fiber and less fat and sugar than pastry or snack cakes. Nuts and dried fruit are higher in calories but are also nutritious and keep well.

Women who bring lunches from home have endless possibilities. It is worth investing in a wide-mouth insulated container for carrying hot—or cold—soups and chowders, stews, salads and interesting leftovers. Sandwich fillings can be prepared at night so they are ready to spread in the morning. A food processor or blender makes it easy to transform poultry, fish or meat left from dinner into a good lunch. Just blend or process the dinner item with some yogurt, a vegetable, perhaps, and seasonings. A few possibilities include chicken with celery and tarragon or with cucumber, curry powder and peanuts; fish with carrots and dill; cottage cheese with green or red peppers, scallions and celery; beef with celery and mustard; and beans with peppers and chili powder. Use different kinds of whole grain breads and rolls to add more variety. Once you get started, the possibilities are endless - just let your imagination go!

Eating in restaurants

Nutritional considerations in choosing meals in restaurants are really the same as those recommended for planning meals at home: eat a variety of foods, including liberal amounts of fiber, green and yellow vegetables, and fruits and vegetables which are rich in vitamin C; and limit the amounts of fat, especially saturated fat and cholesterol; salt; sugar and smoked and cured foods.

The biggest problem most women have when work or travel schedules oblige them to do a lot of eating in restaurants is that they tend to eat more and higher calorie foods and gain weight as a result. The following suggestions on applying nutritional guidelines to menu choices should be helpful.

Breakfast

It is very easy to eat much larger, richer breakfasts in a restaurant than at home. All of the time-consuming prepared dishes are just as readily available as a bowl of cereal, and cream may be more readily available than low fat milk. Fresh fruit and juices are always on the menu and are a good way to start the meal. Whole grain cereals are another good choice as are yogurt or cottage cheese, which are beginning to appear in the morning. Most restaurants have cottage cheese in the kitchen and might be happy to serve it if requested even if it is not listed on the menu.

If you order toast or English muffins, it's a good idea to ask that they be served dry. Even if you use butter or margarine, the amount you spread is probably less than the cook would slather on in the restaurant kitchen. Muffins—bran, corn, blueberry or whatever - are lower in fat and calories than are croissants and other types of breakfast pastry.

Skim or low fat milk may or may not be available, but whole milk always is and can be requested to replace the cream that is often served with coffee or tea. It is worth asking for skim or low fat milk first. Restaurants respond to their customers' wishes and if enough patrons request the lower fat products restaurants will begin to accommodate them.

Lunch and dinner

Choosing an appetizer is usually easy. Fresh fruit, juice or a seafood cocktail would fit nutritional criteria quite nicely. Clear or broth-based soups are another possibility, although they may be too salty for women who need to be particularly careful about their salt intake.

Good selections among main courses include fish, poultry or meat which is roasted, broiled, grilled or baked, in other words, not fried. If you are seriously limiting your fat consumption, ask to have broiled foods prepared and served *dry*; some restaurants serve broiled fish, for example, swimming in a pond of melted butter.

Among vegetables and accompaniments, it's wise to avoid those which are fried or richly sauced. Baked potatoes appear on many menus; ask to have your potato served plain so that you can control the amount of butter or sour cream which goes on it.

Salads are always good, whether as a side dish or as the main meal. The continuing growth of salad bars attests to their popularity. Be careful, though, about falling into the trap of thinking that a meal chosen from the salad bar is automatically low fat and low calorie. That's true of the fresh vegetables but not of grated cheese, bacon bits, nuts, seeds, croutons and dressings, all of which should be used most judiciously. Fresh lemon juice or vinegar can season a salad with no added fat. When the salad is served from the kitchen, you can request vinegar or a wedge of lemon instead of a regular dressing. If you choose to have the dressing, ask to have it served on the side so that you can decide how much to use. Restaurant kitchens are frequently over-generous in their addition of dressing to a salad.

The dessert menu often presents the greatest challenge to the health-conscious woman. While we all recognize that everyone occasionally succumbs to gooey chocolate temptation, there are other possibilities. Fresh fruit is the most obvious choice. Fruit cup or melon may be listed as an appetizer rather than dessert on the menu but will be served for dessert if requested. Sorbets and sherbets have come into fashion in many places and are another good selection. Another option is to skip the dessert entirely and finish the meal with a cup of tea or coffee. Many restaurants now offer freshly brewed decaffeinated coffee which tastes just as good as the regular kind. And, just as at breakfast, you can always ask for milk instead of cream with your beverage.

These suggestions imply that you know what is in a dish when you order it. If the menu is in a foreign language or is unclear about how something is prepared, what ingredients are used, whether vegetables are buttered or anything else you want to know, a question to the server will get you the information. There is no need to be hesitant about asking for information about the food you are ordering.

Fast food restaurants

Fast food restaurants sometimes offer great convenience, especially when time is at a premium. Their drawback lies in their limited menus, which tend to be heavily weighted with fried foods. Fortunately, the trend is towards expanding menus; and even now many fast food establishments offer fruit juices and salad bars to their customers in addition to the standard burgers and French fries. As one would expect, the fried items are highest in fat and calories. Thus, contrary to the general rule of fish being lower in fat than red meat, a fast food (fried) fish sandwich is fatter than a burger, a fact worth bearing in mind when choosing a fast meal.

Drinks

A premeal cocktail is often part of dining out. The calories in alcoholic drinks can come from the liquor itself or the mixer. In the first case, the alcohol itself is the main source of calories so the concentration of alcohol, or proof, is a guide to caloric density. Table wines are the lowest, at about 85 calories per 3 ½-ounce glass. Fortified wines such as sherry and port are somewhat higher, about 140 calories in the same amount. Distilled liquors range from 100 to 135 calories per 1½-ounce jigger. Twelve ounces of beer average 175 calories.

Club soda or water are calorie-free mixers. (A spritzer of wine and club soda is a pleasant, relatively low calorie drink.) Other mixers add calories in proportion to their sweetness.

In addition to the drink itself, snacks served with it can add calories and fat. One tablespoon of peanuts, not a very large amount, contains 7 grams of fat and provides 85 calories.

Exercise

The effects of traveling and eating in restaurants on weight and nutrition are often compounded by decreased physical activity. Awareness is the first step in counteracting the tendency to get less exercise when away from home. The next step is to plan for some activity each day.

The hotel or motel where you stay may have a swimming pool or health club for its guests. Be prepared to take advantage of them by packing a swimsuit as routinely as you pack your toothbrush. If the hotel does not offer exercise facilities, its personnel may be able to advise you about nearby resources.

You could also look up YWCAs and health clubs in the local telephone book. Many of them offer a single admission to non-members from out-of-town.

If scheduling is a problem or these types of activity don't appeal to you, then plan time for a run or brisk walk at some point in the day. Ask at the hotel desk about safe and pleasant routes to take.

As in any discussion of physical activity, the point here is not what you do but that you *do something*. Traveling is a part of many women's lives; it may be frequent or occasional, enjoyable or stressful, comfortably paced or hectic. Whichever it is, it is part of a woman's reality and should not keep her from maintaining routines which promote her health and fitness.

SUGGESTIONS FOR FURTHER READING

1. Food and Nutrition Board, National Research Council: Recommended Dietary Allowances, 9th revised edition, Washington, D.C., National Academy of Sciences, 1980.
    This is the official publication of the RDAs. The presentation is intended for professionals and is rather technical but may be of interest to some readers.

2. Freydberg, Nicholas A. and Willis A. Gortner: The Food Additives Book, New York, Bantam Books, 1982.
    This book describes common food additives, explains their functions and rates their safety. It also lists brand name foods and the additives in them.

3. Hess, Mary Abbot and Anne Elise Hunt: Pickles and Ice Cream: The Complete Guide to Nutrition During Pregnancy, New York, McGraw Hill Book Co., 1982.
    In an easy, chatty style, the authors explain in detail the nutritional needs of the pregnant woman and offer sound, practical advice.

4. Katzen, Mollie: The Moosewood Cookbook, Berkeley, CA, The Ten Speed Press, 1977.
    "Moosewood's" vegetarian recipes are good enough to make this book a favorite of meat-eaters as well.

5. Kraus, Barbara: Calorie Guide to Brand Name and Basic Foods, New York, The New American Library, 1984.
   A widely distributed paperback, this is a ready reference for calorie counters.

6. Messinger, Maire: The Breastfeeding Book, New York, Van Nostrand Reinhold Co., 1982.
   This is a beautifully illustrated, practical handbook for women who plan to breastfeed or want more information to make their choice about infant feeding.

7. Notelovitz, Morris and Marsha Ware: Stand Tall! The Informed Woman's Guide to Preventing Osteoporosis, Gainesville, FL, Triad Publishing Co., 1982.
   Osteoporosis is explained in clear detail, with emphasis on strategies for its prevention.

8. Pennington, Jean A. T. and Helen Nichols Church: Food Values of Portions Commonly Used, 13th edition, New York, Harper and Row, 1980.
   This book of tables is less convenient to use than Kraus (Reference 5) but includes data on protein, fat, carbohydrate, vitamins and minerals in addition to calories.

9. Robertson Laurel, Carol Flinders and Bronwen Godfrey: Laurel's Kitchen: A Handbook for Vegetarians, Berkeley, CA, Nilgiri Press, 1976. (Also available in soft cover)
   Laurel's Kitchen is the best single resource for vegetarians—it combines sound nutrition information with excellent recipes.

10. Satter, Ellyn: Child of Mine: Feeding with Love and Good Sense, Palo Alto, CA, Bull Publishing Co., 1983.
    Satter begins with the mother's diet during pregnancy and continues through the child's third year. Her approach is informative and realistic.

11. Smith, Nathan J.: Food for Sport, Palo Alto, CA, Bull Publishing Co., 1976.
    For athletes, coaches and trainers, this book has all of the information they need on nutrition and athletics.

INDEX

"t" following a page number indicates tabular material.

Acid, conversion of sugar to, dental caries and, 6–7
Acne, 52
Additives, compounds used as, 119
   regulation of, 119–120
   safety of, suggestions for decisions on, 120–121
Adolescence, eating patterns during, 50–51
   growth during, 49
   nutrition in, importance of, 52–53
   nutritional needs during, 50
   pregnancy during, nutritional needs in, 53–55
Adrenalin, 20
Adulthood, nutritional needs during, 57–64
Aging, energy requirements in, 79–80
   mineral requirements in, 80
Alcohol(s), and calcium balance, 83
   as source of energy, 9
   in cocktails, 148–149
   sugar, 8
   use of, 9–10
      and health, 131
      during pregnancy, 72–73
Alcoholism, 10
American Heart Association, fat intake and, 17
Amino acids, essential, 22
   in proteins, 19
   non-essential, 22
   sources of, 22

Anemia, "sports", 88–89
Angina pectoris, 15
Anorexia nervosa, 51–52, 63–64
Antibodies, 20
Aspartame, 9
Atherosclerosis, 14–15
Athletes, carbohydrate loading by, 90–91
   eating on day of event by, 91–92
   exercise of, and nutrient needs, 87–89
   in training, diet for, 90
   protein needs of, 21–22

B-complex vitamins, 26
   and exercise, 88
   functions of, 27
   in pregnancy, 68
Basal metabolic rate (BMR), 98
Basal metabolism, energy expenditure for, 97–98
Beverage(s), alcoholic, calories in, 148–149
   electrolyte, 89
   in meal planning, 139
Bingeing and purging, 64
Blood pressure, sodium and, 41–42
Body weight. *See* Weight(s)
Bone(s), health, calcium and, 58–59
   exercise and, 60, 83–84
   loss, in osteoporosis, 81–82
   mechanical loading of, 83–84
Breakfast, in restaurant, suggestions for, 146–147
   menus for, 139–140

153

Breastfeeding, advantages of, 76
  eating pattern for, 77
  for working mothers, 76–77
  guidance for, 77–78
Broccoli quiche, 140
Budget, food, 121
Bulimia, 64
Buttermilk, 138
Buying. *See* Food buying

Caffeine, and calcium balance, 83
  intake, during pregnancy, 72
  in premenstrual syndrome, 61
Calcium, absorption of, estrogen and, 82–83
  and bone health, 58–59
  balance, high protein diet and, 24
  continuing need for, 37
  functions of, 35–36, 37–40
  intake, osteoporosis and, 58–59
  Recommended Dietary Allowances of, 59
  requirements, 40
    during pregnancy, 69
    in aging, 80
    of vegetarians, 112–113
  sources of, 37, 59
  value of foods, 59
  vegetable sources of, 112
Calcium supplements, 60
Calorie(s), and supplements, 103
  as unit of measurement, 96
  cutting of, in food preparation, 102–103
  dietary, and protein requirements, 21
  food preparation and, 137
  in alcohol, 9, 10
  in weight control program, 100
  increasing of, in underweight, 104–105
  intake, carbohydrates and, 3
  menus to increase and decrease, 105–106
  requirements, during pregnancy, 67, 68
    during training, 90
  value of foods, addition to, in preparation, 100
    components of foods and, 99
    taste and feel in assessment of, 99–100

Cancer, dietary factors and, studies of, 131
  dietary fat and, 17–18
  vitamins and, 32–33
Canned foods, storage of, 135
Canning of foods, 118
Carbohydrate loading, by athletes, 90–91
Carbohydrate(s), 3–10
  absorption of, 4
  and dental caries, 6–7
  classes of, 3
  daily requirements for, 4
  during training, 90
  energy value of, 5
  function of, 4
  nutritional value of, 5–6
Caries, dental. *See* Dental caries
Carotene, 26
  and cancer, 33
Cereals, enrichment of, 123
  in diet, recommendations for, 134
  prices of, 123
Cheeses, choosing of, 124
Chicken parmesan, low fat, 142
Cholesterol, 12
  and cardiovascular health, 15–16
  in foods, 16t
  limitation of, 132
Clostridium botulinum, nitrates and, 120
Cold, common, vitamins and, 32
Constipation, during pregnancy, 75
Containers, food, marking of, 136
Contraceptives, nutritional needs in use of, 63
Convenience foods, cost of, 124–125
  definition of, 124
Corn sweeteners, consumption of, 7
Cured foods, recommendations on, 131
Curing of foods, 118

Dairy products, buying of, 124
  in diet, recommendations for, 134–135
  low-calorie, substitution of, 103
Deficiency diseases, studies of, 130–131
Dehydration of foods, 117–118
Delaney Amendment, 119–120

Dental caries, carbohydrates and, 6–7
　development of, 6
　prevention of, 7
Desserts, in restaurant, 148
Diarrhea, dieter's, 8
Diet, and heart disease, 15–16
　and skin, 52
　during training, 90
　high protein, cautions in, 23–24
　in premenstrual syndrome, 61–62
　recommendations, applications of, 133–134
　vegetarian. See Vegetarian diet(s)
Diet diary, as tool for changing diet, 101
　recording in, 101
　to realize situations leading to eating, 101–102
Dieter's diarrhea, 8
Dinner, in restaurant, suggestions for, 147–148
　menus for, 141–143
Disaccharides, 3
Disease(s), deficiency, studies of, 130–131
　dietary advice to prevent, 130
　prevention, vitamins and, 32–33
　studies of, dietary advice and, 130–131
Dolomite, 40
Dry foods, storage of, 135–136

Eating, at job, 145–146
　away from home, 145–149
　in restaurants, 146–148
Eating disorders, 51–52, 63–64
Eating habits, changing of, for weight control, 101–102
　in "morning sickness", 74
　in premenstrual syndrome, 61–62
　recommendations for, 133–134
　during adolescence, 50–51
　during breastfeeding, 77
　pre-event, by athletes, 91–92
Eggplant, baked stuffed, meatless, 141–142
Electrolyte beverage(s), 89
Energy, alcohol as source of, 9
　balance, weight control and, 96–97

　body use of, functions requiring, 97–98
　carbohydrates and, 3, 5
　consumption, and energy expenditure, 96–97
　fats as source of, 14
　protein and, 20–21
　requirements, during pregnancy, 67–68
　　during training, 90
　　in aging, 79–80
　sources of, in vegetarian diets, 110–111
　value, of body fat, 97
　　of foods, 99–100
Enzymes, 20
Estrogen, levels of, calcium absorption and, 82–83
Exercise(s), and bone health, 60, 83–84
　and nutrient needs, 87–89
　and nutrition, 87
　away from home, 149
　during pregnancy, 67–68
　in premenstrual syndrome, 62–63
　water loss in, 89

Fast food restaurants, menus in, 148
Fat(s), 11–18
　and oils, 11–12
　body, energy value of, 97
　body percentage of, 14
　consumption, and metabolism, 15
　　recommendations on, 131–132, 135
　content of foods, and calorie value, 99
　dietary, and cancer, 17–18
　　and heart disease, 14–17
　digestion of, 12–13
　food preparation and, 137
　functions of, 14
　in foods, 13–14, 13t
　nutritional contributions of, 14
　refraining from adding, in food preparation, 102
　removal of, 103
　sources of, 11, 13–14, 13t
　subcutaneous, measurement of, 94

Fatty acid(s), 11–12
  monounsaturated, 12
  polyunsaturated, 12
  saturated, 11–12
  unsaturated, 12
Fetal alcohol syndrome, 73
Fiber, 3, 4–5
  dietary content of, and disease, 5
    recommendations on, 132
  importance of, 5
  in vegetarian diets, 113
  sources of, 5
Fish, baked, low fat, 142
  buying of, 124
Flour(s), whole grain, 135
  for baking, 138
Fluid(s), intake, during and after athletic event, 92
  in breastfeeding, 77
  retention, during pregnancy, 67
Fluoridation, 43
Fluoride, 42–43
Fluorine, 42–43
Food additives. See Additives
Food and Drug Administration, food additives and, 119
  saccharin and, 8
Food buying, economy in, 121–122
  of fruits and vegetables, 122
  of grains and cereals, 122–123
Food groups, as guide to meal planning, 129
  four, 129
    criticism of, 130
Food market, woman in, 115–125
Food package, information on, 115–117
Food processing, 117–118
Food storage, 135–136
Food(s), aversions, during pregnancy, 76
  calorie value of, addition to, in preparation, 100
  components of foods and, 99
  taste and feel in assessment of, 99–100
  choices, recommendations for, 134–135
  variety in, 120–121
  convenience, cost of, 124–125
    definition of, 124
  cravings, during pregnancy, 75–76
  energy value of, 99–100
  excesses, avoiding of, and health, 130–132
  "imitation", 116
  "natural" and "processed", 117–119
  preparation, 136–138
    cutting calories in, 102–103
  products, comparing of, nutrition labels and, 117
  specific dynamic action of, energy expenditure and, 98
Freeze-dried foods, 118
Freezing of foods, 118
Frozen foods, quality of, maintenance of, 118
Fructose, 3
Fruits, buying of, 122
  in diet, recommendations for, 134
  in healthy desserts, 138

Glucose, 3
Glycogen, 4
Glycogen loading, by athletes, 90–91
Grading of foods, 122
Grain flour(s), 135
  for baking, 138
Grain products, choosing of, 122–123
  enrichment of, 123
  in diet, recommendations for, 134
Grains, and legumes, combining of, 109–110
  minerals in, 41
  value of, 109
GRAS list, 119
Growth, during adolescence, 49
Growth hormone, 20

Haddock, baked, 142
Health, promotion of, avoiding excesses and, 130–132
Heart disease, cholesterol and, 15–16
  diet and, 15–16
  dietary fat and, 14–17
Heartburn, during pregnancy, 75
Heat, to preserve foods, 118
Heavy metals, 40

Height-weight table(s), 94, 95t
Hemoglobin, 20
Hormones, 20
Hypertension, sodium intake and, 41–42

"Imitation", on food label, 116
Indigestion, during pregnancy, 74–75
Ingredients, on food packages, 115–116
    standards of identity and, 116
Insulin, 20
Insurance industry, height-weight standards developed by, 94, 95
Intrauterine contraceptive devices, side effects of, 63
Iron, absorption of, 37
    deficiency, 37
    exercise and, 88–89
    in diet, increasing of, 58
    in sweeteners and other foods, 6t
    Recommended Dietary Allowances of, 37, 58
    requirements, during pregnancy, 69
    in adulthood, 57–58
    in aging, 80
    sources of, for vegetarians, 113

Job, eating at, 145–146
Joule, definition of, 96

Kilocalorie, definition of, 96

Labels, food, information on, 115–117
Lactase deficiency, 4
Lactose, absorption of, 4
Lead, 40
Legumes, and grains, combining of, 109–110
    in vegetarian diets, 109–110
Lipids, 11
Lipoproteins, high density, 13
    low density, 13
Liquid meals, for athletes, 92
List, for food shopping, 121–122
Lunch, at workplace, suggestions for, 146
    in restaurant, 147–148
    menus for, 140–141

Mannitol, 8
Margarine, 137
Market, food, woman in, 115–125
Meal pattern(s). *See* Menu(s)
Meal planning, applying recommendations to, 132–134
    benefits of, 121
    food groups in, 129
        criticism of, 130
    menus for, 138–143
    nutrition labels and, 117
    nutritional adequacy and, 127–130
    Recommended Dietary Allowances and, 128
Meals, liquid, for athletes, 92
Meat(s), buying of, 123–124
    grading of, 123
Meatloaf, low fat, 142
Menopause, symptoms of, 81
Menu(s), breakfast, 139–140
    dinner, 141–143
    for pregnant adolescent, 53–55
    in fast food restaurants, 148
    in meal planning, 138–143
    in pregnancy, 70–72
    in premenstrual syndrome, 62
    lunch, 140–141
    to increase and decrease caloric value, 105–106
Mercury, 40
Metals, heavy, 40
Milk, and milk substitutes, 137–138
    buying of, 124
    dry, 124
    for vegetarians, 109
    in diet, recommendations for, 134
    powdered skim, increasing calcium value of, 137–138
Milkshake, breakfast, 139
Mineral(s), 35–43
    deficiencies, 37
    functions of, 35–36, 36, 38–39t
    in foods, 40–41
    in human skeleton, 35
    requirements, 36
        during pregnancy, 68–69
        in aging, 80
    sources of, for vegetarians, 112–113
    trace, 36

Index

Monosaccharides, 3
Multivitamin-mineral supplements, calories and, 103
Myocardial infarction, 15

"Natural" foods, 117–119
Nausea, during pregnancy, 74
Nitrates, in foods, 120
Nutrient(s), essential, 1–46
   need for, during pregnancy, 67
   exercise and, 87–89
   on food labels, 116–117
   preservation of, in food preparation, 136–137
   sources, during pregnancy, 69–72
Nutrition, exercise and, 87
   in special interests, 85–113
Nutrition information, on food packages, 116–117
Nutritional needs, during adolescence, 50
   in adulthood, 57–64
   in aging, 80–81
   in pregnancy, during adolescence, 53–55
   in use of contraceptive devices, 63
Nuts, storage of, 135

Obesity, conference on (1975), height-weight guidelines from, 94–95, 95t
   risks associated with, 95
Oils, fats and, 11
   vegetable, 12
Oral contraceptives, side effects of, 63
Osteoporosis, 40, 81–84
   bone loss in, 81–82
   calcium intake and, 58–59, 80
   dynamic state of skeleton and, 81–82
   prevention of, estrogen replacement in, 83
   increased calcium intake in, 83
   nutrition in, 82
Overfat, definition of, 94
Overweight, definition of, 94

Package, food, information on, 115–117

Phosphorus, functions of, 35–36
Physical activity, benefits of, 98
   choice of, factors influencing, 98
   energy expenditure and, 98
   increasing of, upon ceasing smoking, 104
   "self-monitoring" of, 102
   walking as, 98–99
Phytate, 113
Plaque, in atherosclerosis, 14–15
Pregnancy, 65–78
   common problems during, handling of, 74–78
   constipation during, 75
   during adolescence, nutritional needs in, 53–55
   energy requirements during, 67–68
   fluid retention during, 67
   food cravings and aversions during, 75–76
   heartburn and indigestion during, 74–75
   items to avoid during, 72–74
   nausea and vomiting during, 74
   nutrient sources during, 69–72
   protein requirements during, 68
   vitamin and mineral requirements during, 68–69
   weight changes in, division of, 66
   weight gain during, 66–67
Premenstrual syndrome, 60–62
   dietary changes in, 61–62
   exercise in, 62–63
   symptoms of, 61
"Processed" foods, 117–119
Protein(s), 19–24
   amino acids in, 19
   and calcium balance, 83
   and energy, 20–21
   as enzymes, 20
   as hormones, 20
   complete, 22
   diet high in, calcium balance and, 24
   cautions in, 23–24
   elements in, 19
   extra, 23–24
   food, in diet, recommendations for, 134
   sources of, 123–124

functions of, 19–20
  in cells and tissues, 20
  in foods, 22–23, 23t
  in vegetarian diets, 109–110
  incomplete, 22
  requirements, 23
    athletics and, 21–22
    conditions increasing, 21
    dietary calories and, 21
    during pregnancy, 68
    exercise and, 88
    factors determining, 21
  vegetable sources of, 109
Pyridoxine, 27

Quiche, broccoli, 140

Radiation, in food preservation, 119
Recommended Dietary Allowances, and minimal daily requirements, 128
  background and intent of, 128
  expansion of uses of, 128
  of calcium, 59
  of iron, 37, 58
  of vitamins, 31
  on food labels, 116–117
  usefulness of, limitation of, 128–129
Restaurants, choosing meals in, 146–148
  fast food, 148
Riboflavin, sources of, for vegetarians, 112
Rice, and rice mixes, 123

Saccharin, Food and Drug Administration and, 8
  risks and benefits associated with, 8–9
Salads, low fat/low calorie, in restaurant, 147–148
Salt, intake, decreasing of, 137
  in premenstrual syndrome, 61
Selenium, 42
Serving size, in nutrition information, 116
Shopping, planning in, 121–122
Skin, diet and, 52
Skinfold calipers, for fat measurement, 94
Smoked foods, recommendations on, 132

Smoking, and weight, 104
  effects of, pregnancy and, 73–74
Snacks, foods for, 50
  nutritious, at job, 145
  for weight gain, 105
Sodium, and blood pressure, 41–42
  intake, during pregnancy, 69
  recommendations on, 132
  requirements, in exercise, 89
  sources of, 41
Sodium chloride, 41
Sodium nitrate, in cured meat and fish, 120
Sorbitol, 8
Standards of identity, 116
Starches, 3
  as simple sugars, 3
Sterols, 12
Sucrose, 3
Sugar alcohols, 8
Sugar substitutes, 8–9
Sugar(s), 3
  absorption of, 4
  concentrated, before athletic events, 92
  consumption of, 7
    cutting down on, 7
  conversion to acid, dental caries and, 6–7
  differences between, 5–6
  forms of, 5
  reduction of, in recipes, 103
  simple, 3
Sweeteners, 5–6
  corn, consumption of, 7
  iron content of, 6t
  non-caloric, 8–9
Sweets, in diet, recommendations on, 135

Thirst, 46
Tobacco, use of, during pregnancy, 73–74
Trace minerals, 36
Traveling, exercise while, 149

U.S. Food and Drug Administration. *See* Food and Drug Administration
Underweight, evaluation of, 104
  increasing of weight in, 104–105
  snacking in, 105

Vegans, 108
Vegetable oils, 12
Vegetables, as source of proteins, 109
  buying of, 122
  cruciferous, 132
  in diet, recommendations for, 134
Vegetarian diet(s), adequacy of, 108–109
  energy sources in, 110–111
  minerals in, 112–113
  protein in, 109–110
  vitamins in, 111–112
Vegetarian(s), calcium requirements of, 112–113
  lacto, 108
  ovo-lacto, 108
  reasons for becoming, 108
  strict, 108
Vegetarianism, contemporary, 108
  history of, 107–108
Vitamin A, 26
  and acne, 52
  and cancer, 33
  in pregnancy, 68
  sources of, 132
Vitamin B12, sources of, for vegetarians, 112
Vitamin C, 26
  and cancer, 33
  and common cold, 32
  in pregnancy, 68–69
  sources of, 132
Vitamin D, 26
  and calcium absorption, 83
  in pregnancy, 69
  sources of, for vegetarians, 111
Vitamin E, 27
Vitamin K, 27
Vitamin supplements, 32
  calories and, 103
Vitamin(s), 25–33
  and disease prevention, 32–33
  B-complex. See B-complex vitamins
  deficiency(ies), 31–32
    subclinical, 31–32
  definition of, 25
  fat-soluble, absorption of, 26
  food preparation and, 136
  food storage and, 135
  functions of, 27, 28–30t
  in premenstrual syndrome, 62
  in vegetarian diets, 111–112
  naming of, 25
  Recommended Dietary Allowances of, 31
  requirements, 27–31
    during pregnancy, 68–69
  solubility and toxicity of, 26–27
  water-soluble, absorption of, 26
Vomiting, during pregnancy, 74

Walking, as physical activity, 98–99
Water, content of food, and calorie value, 99
  during and after athletic event, 92
  functions of, 45
  loss, determination of, 89
    in exercise, 89
    in weight loss schemes, 97
  requirements, 45–46
  sources of, 46
Weight(s), and fat, distinction between, 94
  as guide to nutrient needs, 88
  concern with, during adolescence, 50–51
  in adulthood, 93–106
  control, by adolescents, 51
    energy balance and, 96–97
    strategies for, 100–102
  desirable, calculation of, 94
  choosing of, 93–94
  confusion concerning, 93
  estimates of, purposes of, 95–96
  maintenance of, 131
  gain, during pregnancy, 66–67
  ideal body, protein need and, 21
  smoking and, 104
Workplace, eating at, 145–146

Yogurt, uses of, 137

Zinc, 37
  sources of, for vegetarians, 113